Hepatotoxicity

Edited by Costin-Teodor Streba,
Ion Rogoveanu and Cristin Constantin Vere

Published in London, United Kingdom

Hepatotoxicity
http://dx.doi.org/10.5772/intechopen.98062
Edited by Costin-Teodor Streba, Ion Rogoveanu and Cristin Constantin Vere

Contributors
Umar Hayat, Hafiz Zubair, Muhammad Farhan, Ahmad Haris, Ali Siddiqui, Nida Mirza, Ihegboro Godwin, Chimaobi James Ononamadu, Debnarayan Dutta, Yarlagadda Sreenija, Youcai Tang, Xuecui Yin, Yuying Ma, Rahmat Adetutu Adisa, Lateef Adegboyega Sulaimon, Costin-Teodor Streba, Victor-Mihai Sacerdotianu, Ion Rogoveanu, Liliana Streba, Cristin Constantin Vere

First published in London, United Kingdom, 2022 by IntechOpen
IntechOpen is the global imprint of INTECHOPEN LIMITED, registered in England and Wales, registration number: 11086078, 5 Princes Gate Court, London, SW7 2QJ, United Kingdom

British Library Cataloguing-in-Publication Data
A catalogue record for this book is available from the British Library

Additional hard and PDF copies can be obtained from orders@intechopen.com

Hepatotoxicity
Edited by Costin-Teodor Streba, Ion Rogoveanu and Cristin Constantin Vere
p. cm.
Print ISBN 978-1-80355-780-9
Online ISBN 978-1-80355-781-6
eBook (PDF) ISBN 978-1-80355-782-3

Meet the editors

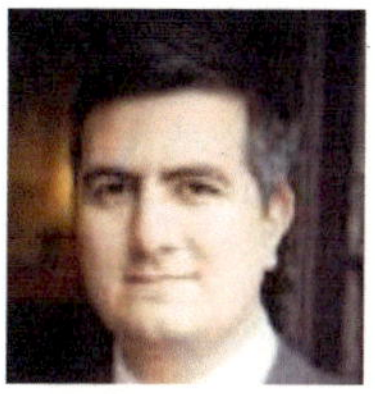

Costin Teodor Streba, MD, Ph.D., MSc, is a professor at the University of Medicine and Pharmacy of Craiova, Romania, and a member of the university's Research Center of Gastroenterology and Hepatology of Craiova. He has extensive research experience in liver and pancreatic disease diagnostics and training in histological image analysis. He specialized in devising medical-oriented diagnostic systems for liver malignancies that integrate interpretation and computer-aided quantification of various imaging and clinical data. Dr. Teodor has published extensively on innovative diagnostic techniques in gastroenterology.

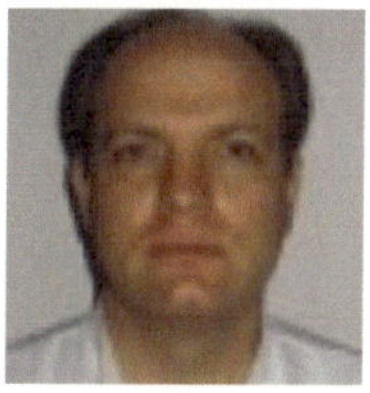

Cristin Constantin Vere, MD, Ph.D., MSc, is a Professor of Gastroenterology at the University of Medicine and Pharmacy of Craiova, Romania, and one of the founding members of the university's Research Center of Gastroenterology and Hepatology of Craiova. His research interests span from neuroimmune mechanisms of liver disease to novel diagnostic techniques in gastroenterology. Pioneering the introduction of wireless video capsules in Romania, Dr. Constantin established a dynamic team of Ph.D. students and full-time scientists specialized in both medical sciences and bioinformatics. He has published extensively on hepatology and the complex integrative mechanisms that form the basis for this pathology.

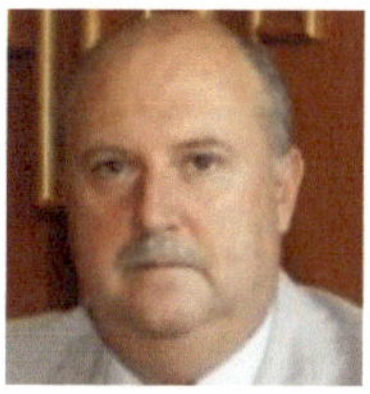

Ion Rogoveanu , MD, Ph.D., MSc, is a Professor of Gastroenterology at the University of Medicine and Pharmacy of Craiova, Romania, and one of the founding members of the university's Research Center of Gastroenterology and Hepatology of Craiova. Mentoring a team of dedicated doctors and managing the curricular and scientific activities of the university as rector, Dr. Ion is currently one of the lead authorities in ultrasound and power Doppler US, coordinating postgraduate courses for the past 10 years. His most prestigious publications are on the prevention, diagnosis, and treatment of hepatocellular carcinoma (HCC) and various liver diseases.

Contents

Preface

The liver is an essential organ with important roles in metabolism, digestion, and immunity. When the liver is too injured and its role cannot be fulfilled at a minimum required level, liver failure occurs and all aforementioned processes are disturbed with a negative impact on patients. This stage is associated with important morbidity, and mortality, and has limited therapeutical resources; sometimes liver transplant is the only remaining option. Therefore, every potentially harmful agent for the liver must be avoided.

However, some of these agents are deliberately recommended for their therapeutic benefit in certain diseases and liver injury occurs as an adverse effect, which makes it difficult for the prescribing physician. The medical option must be clearly explained to patients who must understand why the treatment is important and that the drugs may have an unwanted secondary effect on the liver. Some patients are diagnosed with an incurable disease and the only role of the drug is to prolong survival for an unknown variable period. For these patients, the possibility that a liver injury can occur during therapy may influence their decision to give consent because it is hard to admit that a treatment indicated to reduce the harmful impact of one disease can lead to the appearance of a new disease. In these cases, the risks and benefits of the potential hepatotoxic therapeutical agents must be carefully analyzed by one or more experienced physicians and a decision individualized to the patient must be made.

Multiple medical specialties, especially oncology, rheumatology, and gastroenterology, use therapeutic regimens that may contain agents that can have negative repercussions on liver functions. As such, this book provides comprehensive information on hepatotoxicity with the common purpose of better understanding the liver injury that can occur due to certain drugs prescribed for multiple health problems. Chapters present the latest data in terms of epidemiology, pathogenesis, clinical manifestations, diagnostic methods, and treatment options for the topics addressed in this book.

This book is a useful resource for treating physicians across various specialties as well as physicians in training.

Costin-Teodor Streba, Ion Rogoveanu and Cristin Constantin Vere
University of Medicine and Pharmacy of Craiova,
Craiova, Romania

Section 1

Hepatotoxicity Induced by Drugs

Chapter 1

Drug-Induced Hepatotoxicity

Godwin Okwudiri Ihegboro and Chimaobi James Ononamadu

Abstract

This chapter aims at discussing the consequential effects of drug-induced hepatotoxicity on man. The liver carries out drug detoxification among other roles, but sometimes, drug toxicity can occur caused by either medication overdose or imbalance drug metabolic reactions (Phase 1 & 2), resulting in the formation of reactive (toxic) metabolites (electrophilic compounds or free radicals) that binds covalently to hepatocytes, leading to liver injury/diseases like acute and chronic hepatitis, cholestasis, steatosis among others. Mitochondrial dysfunction, oxidative stress and lipid peroxidation are some of the mechanisms of liver injury. Furthermore, drug hepatotoxicity results in hepatocellular, gastroenterological, cholestatic as well as immunological disorders. The clinical manifestations of drug toxicity arise from the abnormalities observed in liver's biochemical and molecular indicators. Our findings, revealed that in the event of liver injury, liver function indices like aspartate and alanine aminotransferases, ALP (alkaline phosphatase) and gamma glutamyl transferase (GGT) activities, intracellular calcium (Ca^{2+}) and lipid peroxidation increases whereas indices of oxidative stress such as glutathione and its allies, catalase and superoxide dismutase activity deplete. At molecular level, the gene expression levels of Bcl-2 mRNA and microRNA genes (miR-122, 192 and 194) reduces while mitochondrial genes (MMP-2 and MMP-9) overexpresses. Since drug abuse is deleterious to human health, therefore, adherence to doctors' prescription guidelines should be followed.

Keywords: liver, hepatotoxic agents, hepatotoxicity, liver indicators, gene expression

1. Introduction

The liver is a reddish-brown multifunctional organ that lies beneath the diaphragm in the abdomen's right upper quadrant and overlies the gallbladder. It performs varieties of biological and metabolic functions, but one significant of them is xenobiotic metabolism/detoxification, in which exogeneous lipophilic xenobiotics (drugs and herbal supplements) are converted to hydrophilic compounds via biochemical processes catalysed by cytochrome P_{450} enzyme systems. The metabolic products obtained are then actively transported by hepatocyte transporter proteins into the plasma or bile for excretion by the kidney or gastrointestinal tract [1, 2]. However, sometimes, these xenobiotics produce reactive (or toxic) metabolites or electrophiles that bind covalently to hepatocytes, resulting to changes in protein conformation, DNA mutation or induce lipid peroxidation respectively, thereby leading to hypersensitivity reaction or liver necrosis. This is known as drug-induced injury (or hepatogenous poisoning, toxic-liver disease, chemical-driven injury). This situation often leads to hospitalisation and/or liver transplantation, depending on the magnitude of the liver injury [3]. There are over 1000 hepatotoxic agents available, however, drugs account for about 20–40% of the cases associated with liver failure/injury [4]. Notably, there are two categories of drug-induced liver injury (DILI) namely: intrinsic (or pharmacological) and idiosyncratic DILI respectively. Intrinsic DILI, refer to a form of liver toxicity caused by a drug in a projectable and dose-dependent manner (e.g. acetaminophen). In this circumstance, liver injury sets-in after an elevated concentration of the drug is attained. On the other hand, idiosyncratic DILI (which occurs relatively), is a non-projectable, non-dose-dependent response to drug and differs in the period of latency (e.g. Trovafloxacin and Troglitazone). It is worthy of note, that approximately 75–80% cases of idiosyncratic reactions end up in death or liver transplantation and as such precautionary measures should be observed in the use of drugs [5, 6]. The dreadful incidences of DILI can be checked by creating drug pharmacovigilant awareness, in which cases of adverse side effects after drug administration should be withdrawn or stopped abruptly to avoid further harm to the body. Besides the harmful effects of acetaminophen (APAP) overdose that has been well documented, studies provide us with wide spectrum of drug inducible agents like, Atypical antipsychotic (AAP), D-galactosamine ((D-GalN)), N-nitrosodiethylamine (NDEA), thioacetamide, Anti- Tuberculosis Drugs (ATD), Anti- Retroviral Drugs (ARDs), Antimalarial Drugs, NSAIDs (Non-Steroidal Anti-inflammatory Drugs), azacytidine, to mention but a few [3]. Therefore, this chapter focuses on discussing the mechanism of action and toxicological implications of drug-induced hepatotoxicity of the aforementioned drugs to human health.

2. Drugs and their role in hepatotoxicity

2.1 Paracetamol

As much as there are several analgesic drugs consumed by man as pain killer agents, paracetamol seems to be the commonly used and contains acetaminophen - the active ingredient, which has been shown to be well-tolerated in prescribed dose but in the event of overdose, liver damage occurs. This is because, acetaminophen metabolism catalysed by cytochrome P_{450} enzymes in the liver produces N-acetyl-p-benzoquineimine (NAPBQI) – a highly reactive (toxic) intermediate metabolite [7]. In the normal sense, this metabolite gets detoxified by glutathione conjugation in phase II reaction. Nevertheless, during acetaminophen's overdose, a high concentration of the toxic metabolite is produced, and thus overwhelms the detoxification process, leading to hepatocellular necrosis. Reports have shown that liver injury caused by this metabolite can be reduced by the administration of acetylcysteine - a precursor of glutathione, by scavenging the toxic metabolite from the system [8].

2.2 Atypical antipsychotic (AAP)

Antipsychotic drugs are detoxified via the cytochrome-P_{450} system in the phase 1 and phase 11 reactions. In its metabolism, the enzyme known as mono-oxygenase converts the drugs into less toxic metabolites through hydrolysis, oxido-reduction and dealkylation processes. However, sometimes, the phase products may display high level of toxicity, hence, phase 11 reaction becomes inevitable. The phase II reaction mainly involves a biochemical process called conjugation reaction which makes use of glucuronic acid, sulphate, acetate, amino acids and glutathione to convert phase 1 products to a more body friendly form and subsequently for excretion. Many antipsychotic drugs beside antisulpride, risperidone, and paliperidone are catabolised primarily via the CYP2D6 and CYP3A4 systems while clozapine and olanzapine use the CYP1A2 system for its drug metabolism. Experimentation shows that antipsychotic drugs potentially damages liver cells through three mechanisms (i) By increasing bile secretion and excretion leading to cholestasis which relates to immune-mediated hypersensitivity (a typical mechanism of chlorpromazine) (ii) Accumulation of toxic or reactive intermediates (or metabolites) that eventually attacks liver cells (iii) By Increasing the risk of metabolic idiosyncratic syndrome leading to high risk of non-alcoholic fatty liver diseases which is typical of olanzapine and clozapine. Indiscriminate consumption of antipsychotic drugs presents some clinical manifestations (or side effects) and this can be encapsulated into four categories namely:

1. Hepatocellular disorder in which hepatic bio-indicators such as aminotransferases, ALP (alkaline phosphatase) and γ-glutamyl transferase (GGT) activities as well as the levels of albumin and total bilirubin are found to increase significantly in the serum.

2. Gastrointestinal disorders ranging from fatigue, appetite loss, excruciating pains in the liver region and epigastric discomfort

3. Cholestasis and steatosis like coloured stool

4. Immunological or hypersensitivity disorders including eosinophilia, anthralgia, rashes, acute liver failure (ALF), auto-immune diseases among others [9, 10].

2.3 D-galactosamine (D-GalN)

Galactosamine, one of the commonly used experimental model for hepatotoxicity study in animals, is an amino sugar derivative found majorly as glycoprotein in living cells. In addition, it forms a component of some hormonal systems like Luteinizing hormone (LH) and Follicle stimulating hormone (FSH) respectively. Biochemical investigation into the hepatotoxic effect of D-galactosamine revealed that it induces liver damage by interfering with the products of galactosamine metabolism via Leloir pathway of galactose metabolism. Firstly, galactosamine is transformed to galactosamine-1-phosphate (Gal-1-P) catalysed by galactokinase while the second phase involves the conversion of galactosaminr-1-phosphate to Uridine diphosphate-galactosamine (UDPG) by galactose uridyltransferase. At low substrate specificity, UDPG inhibits the activity of UDP-galactose-4^1-epimerase, thereby causing a significant accumulation in the hepatic cells and others like UDP-N-acetylglucosamine and UDP-N-acetyl galactosamine with corresponding depletions of uridine triphosphate (UTP), uridine diphosphate (UDP), uridine monophosphate (UMP) as well as uridine diphosphate-glucose (UDP-Glu) and uridine diphosphate-galactose (UDP-Gal), respectively. The outcome of this process then causes the loss of intracellular Ca^{2+} homeostasis, inhibits hepatocyte ATP metabolism and hepatitis which invariably affects cell membrane, inhibits mRNA, protein and nucleic acid biosynthesis. These effects increase protein gene (p53) expression and decreases Bcl-2 mRNA levels in the liver. It is noteworthy, that the hepatoxic action of galactosamine is effective when in combination with lipopolysaccharide (GalN/LPS). This combination induces the Kupffer cells to secrete pro-inflammatory mediators that leads to liver cell apoptosis [11]. Experimental design that involves the treatment of animals with D-GalN alters albumin mRNA, glucose-6-phosphatase, histone-3 mRNA, alpha feto-protein mRNA (αFP mRNA), gamma-glutamyl transpeptidase (GGTP) expressions. Furthermore, it also upregulates expression of tumour nuclear factor (TNF-α mRNA) that has activity of necrotic factor-kappa B (NF- κB10) and alter membrane cofactor protein (MCP-1) level in serum. Also, serum ALT and AST activities increases substantially [12, 13].

2.4 N-nitrosodiethylamine (NDEA)

N-nitrosodiethylamine (NDEA), is a member of the nitrosamine family and are found in various foodstuff and underground water with high nitrate level. It has hepatocarcinogenic property by yielding adducts of DNA carcinogen in the liver and induces hepatic cancer. NDEA's mechanism of hepatic damage is such that after treatment, it stimulates increase in liver mitochondrial transitional permeability (MTP), leading to increase hydrogen peroxide (H_2O_2) production, resulting in peroxidative stress [14, 15]. Alternatively, cytochrome P_{450} activates NDEA, generating reactive electrophilic molecules capable of increasing oxidative stress and liver cytotoxicity and carcinogenicity [16].

2.5 Thioacetamide

Thioacetamide (TAA), is a white crystalline, organosulfur compound with high affinity for water and alcohol. It is chemically designated as C_2H_5NS and generally classified as class 2B human carcinogenic agent. NDEA exhibits wide range of relevance such as serve as sulphide source in the synthesis of compounds (organic and inorganic), controls the deterioration of orange fruits (fungicidal role), precipitates cadmium sulphide from acidic solutions, drug development, pesticide production, serve as cross-linking agent but to mention a few. However, scientific reports documented that long-term oral consumption of TAA causes liver cell adenomas, cholangiomas and hepatocarcinomas as well as affects protein, nuclei acid synthesis and GGTP activity. The bio-transformation of TAA via oxidative bioactivation in the liver microsomes catalysed by flavin-containing mono-oxygenases (FMOs) and cytochrome P450 systems produce two toxic metabolites. Firstly, TAA is catalysed by thioacetamide-S-oxygenase to form a reactive intermediate, thioacetamide-S-oxide (TAASO) adduct through oxidation process, which then induces hepatocytic oxidative stress, resulting to increase in nucleoli and Ca^{2+} concentrations as well as inhibit mitochondrial activity, thereby leading to hepatotoxicity with a resultant effect of centrilobular necrosis. However, the action of CYP2E1 inhibitors (such as 4-methylpyrazole and diallyl sulphide) and TAA, block TAASO toxicity in a relative and absolute manner respectively. The second phase of metabolism involves the conversion of TAASO to thioacetamide-S-S-dioxide ($TAASO_2$ - a reactive species) by the action of thioacetamide-S-oxide-S-oxygenase and then covalently binds with protein and nucleic acid causing hepatotoxicity with consequential effect of liver damage/injury [17, 18]. The characteristic validation of the hepatotoxic effect of TAA includes decrease in microRNA gene expression (miR-122, miR-192 and miR-194) and increase in AST and ALT activities, mitochondrial membrane protein gene expression (MMP-9 and MMP-2) as well as myeloperoxidase, interleukin-10 (IL-10) and tumour nuclear factor (TNFα) respectively [19–21].

2.6 Acetylaminofluorene (AAF)/DEN

This is a fluorine derivative compound with carcinogenic tenacity. Its incorporation in diet and subsequent administration induces increased incidences of liver and urinary bladder carcinomas in animal model. Acetylaminofluorene, a by-product of diethyl nitrosamine (DEN) initiates carcinogenesis by increasing reactive oxygen species (ROS) production and facilitate hyperproliferation [22]. Acetylaminofluorene metabolism by cytochrome P_{450} produces metabolites like 2-aminofluorene (AF), 2-glycoloylamino-fluorene (2-GAF), N-hydroxy-2-acetylaminofluorene (NH-2-AAF), 2-acetylaminofluo-ren-3-,-7-,-9-ol (3-, 7-, 9-hydroxy-AAF) and 2-acetylaminofluoren-9-one (AAF-9-one) respectively and exhibits different toxicity pathway. For instance, N-hydroxy-2-acetylaminofluorene and AAF binds covalently at Carbon - 8th positions in guanine; causing single strand breaks in DNA with resultant effect of severe apoptosis. Sometimes, AAF exposure increases expression of genes implicated in p53-signalling pathway, mRNA genes [encode mitochondria drug resistance proteins (Mdr1b, Mrp1 and Mrp3)] and microRNA genes respectively, thereby resulting in apoptosis [23–25]. Studies showed that at small dose of 2-AAF for long (2.24 or 22.4 mg/kg, 3 times/week for 31 days) or high dose (448 mg/kg BW, i.g., 5 days/week for 8 weeks) produces maximum hepatocellular carcinogenesis through AAF- DNA adducts [26, 27]. Interestingly, lower dose of 2-AAF (50 mg/kg BW, i.p.) was reported to increase lipid peroxidation, deplete GSH level while the activities of glutathione peroxidase (GPx), glutathione reductase (GR), catalase (CAT), and glutathione-S-transferase (GST) were significantly reduced [28].

2.7 Anti- tuberculosis drugs (ATD)

Anti-tubercular drugs are the most auspicious prescription medication used for the treatment of cases of tuberculosis - an infectious disease with high mortality rate [29]. However, long- term administration of anti-tubercular drugs like rifampicin (RIF), isoniazid (INH) and pyrazinamide (PZA) (first line anti-tubercular drugs), significantly increase hepatotoxicity and induces liver injury in mammals [30]. The mechanism that precipitates anti-tubercular drug's liver damage maybe unclear, nevertheless, studies show significant increases in alanine aminotransferase (ALT), aspartate aminotransferase (AST) and alkaline phosphatase (ALP) activities. Furthermore, lipid peroxidation, intracellular calcium (Ca^{2+}) level and $CYP_{450}2EI$ activity also increases while GSH level, GPx and catalase activities decreases [31]. Recently, research shows that acetylators generate high level of acetylated drug which undergo further metabolism to yield other toxic intermediates which causes liver disruption, for instance, Isoniazid acetylation by N-acetyltransferase (NTA2) enzyme produces mono-acetyl hydrazine (MAH) that increases liver toxicity [32]. Notably, polymorphism at gene loci of NTA2, CYP2E1 and GST (detoxifying enzymes) modulate the activities of these enzymes and hence increases the risk of hepatotoxicity [33]. Studies have shown some administrable dose regimen of anti-tubercular drugs that can be used for biochemical evaluation, for example, intraperitoneal administration of 50 mg/kg BW of isoniazid, 100 mg/kg BW of rifampicin and intragastric administration of 350 mg/kg BW of pyrazinamide respectively. Also, when they are in combined form such as INH and RIF as well as INH, RIF and PZA induces hepatotoxicity. This observation was in agreement with previous work as reported by [34] that daily oral administration of isoniazid (15 mg/kg BW), rifampicin (20 mg/kg BW) and pyrazinamide (35 mg/kg BW) in combined form for 45 days, increases malondialdehyde level (MDA).

2.8 Anti- retroviral drugs (ARDs)

The therapeutic action of highly active antiretroviral drugs (HAART) like Protease inhibitors (PI), non-Nucleoside reverse transcriptase inhibitors (nNRTI) and Nucleoside/Nucleotide reverse transcriptase inhibitors (NRTI) used in the management of human immunodeficiency virus (HIV) undergo various pathways, nonetheless, their adverse effects are targeted/localised at the hepatic cells [35, 36]. Take for example, all anti-retroviral therapy-native (ART-naïve) like atazanavir or ritonavir and NRTIs (such as zidovudine or didanosine) alongside N-Apostolova Efavirenz (nNRTI) causes hepatic mitochondrial dysfunction and acute mitotoxic effect and oxidative stress respectively [37, 38]. Furthermore, administration of 50 μM of Efavirenz (EFV) can activate the activities of caspase-3 and caspase −9, trigger apoptotic mitochondrial intrinsic pathway and directly inhibit mitochondrial complex 1 subunit (MC1s) expression [39, 40]. The therapeutic efficacy of antiretroviral drugs is seen when used in combinations such as nNRTI and NRTIs but reports have documented that this combination produces deleterious effects on the mitochondria and also cause hepatic steatosis [41]. Another typical mechanism of action of some antiretroviral drug like stavudine (NRTI) is its ability to arrest cell cycle in growth phase (G1 phase) through upregulation of cyclic-dependent kinase inhibitor (CDKN2A) as well as p21 genes and inhibiting mitochondrial DNA replication [42].

2.9 Anti-malarial drugs

Amodiaquine (an anti-malarial drug) hepatotoxic effect is achieved in humans when it is being oxidised by liver microsomes and peroxidases, produces iminoquinone, (a reactive metabolite) which binds to proteins irreversibly, causing direct liver toxicity by disrupting the hepatocyte function [43].

2.10 Anti-hyperlipidemic drugs

This class of drugs act mainly by hepatocellular or mixed reactions and rarely by cholestatic reaction. The Niacin and Statin are the commonly used drugs in the treatment of hyperlipidemic conditions, however, they have potential to induce liver injury. Studies revealed that the administration of Lovastatin and Simvastatin in animal model (rabbits or Guinea pig) resulted in hepatocellular necrosis while Atorvastatin produced a mixed pattern of liver injury. It is noteworthy, that Simvastatin in combination with other drugs like flutamide, troglitazone and diltiazem gives a more pronounced hepatic effect and this has been attributed to the drug–drug interaction mechanism [1].

2.11 Non-steroidal anti-inflammatory drugs (NSAIDs)

The liver damaging effects of NSAIDs like acetylsalicylic acid ranges from elevated ALT, AST and ALP activities to acute cytolytic, cholestatic or mixed hepatitis as well as increases in bilirubin and prothrombin time. The mechanistic action of NSAID-induced hepatotoxicity is unclear but both intrinsic (Aspirin and phenylbutazone) and idiosyncratic (Ibuprofen, sulindac, phenylbutazone, piroxicam, diclofenac and indomethacin) reactions have been documented [44]. Suggestively, hypersensitivity and metabolic aberrations are thought to responsible for liver injury. Unlike hypersensitivity reactions that are characterised by considerable anti-nuclear factor or anti-smooth muscle antibody titres as well as lymphadenopathy and eosinophilia, metabolic aberrations are caused by genetic polymorphisms, altering susceptibility to variety of drugs [45]. Diclofenac hepatotoxicity in humans and rats, for example, is linked to mitochondrial ATP synthesis impairment and the production of N-5-dihydroxydiclofenac (active metabolites), which causes cytotoxicity. Also, diclofenac-induced liver injury results in mitochondrial transition permeability (MTP), causing ROS formation, protein thiols production, mitochondrial swelling and oxidation of $NADP^+$ (Nicotinamide adenine dinucleotide phosphate) respectively [45].

2.12 Anti-hypertensive drug

This anti-hypertensive drug called methyl dopa metabolises in the liver by Cytochrome P_{450}, however, the oxidative reaction of methyl dopa by CYP_{450} produces superoxide anions (free radicals) to a reactive quinone or semi-quinone that binds tightly to the hepatic cells causing liver injury such as acute/chronic hepatitis and cholestasis with clinical evidence of elevated activities of ALT, AST and ALP respectively in the blood system [1].

2.13 Azacytidine drug

Azacytidine (or Azacitidine), is a pyrimidine nucleoside analogue of cytidine which is metabolised to a triphosphate molecule in the intracellular domain and then introduced into the RNA and DNA molecule firmly held together covalently by DNA methyltransferase 1(DNMT 1) - an enzyme that adds methyl to DNA molecule at the carbon 5 position of cytosine. Azacitidine has an anticancer effect but at low doses, it inhibits DNA methylation resulting in its deactivation leading to DNA hypomethylation shortly after cell division in the absence of DNMT1. The antineoplastic activity of this drug comes from its hypomethylation, leading to tumour suppressor gene (TSG) reactivation which is rapidly lost in myelodysplastic syndrome (MDS) – a disorder associated with clonal haematopoietic stem cell, caused mainly due to ineffective cellular maturation with side effects as peripheral blood cytopenia and abnormalities in functional blood cell. The cytotoxic effect of azacytidine is achieved when the product of its phosphorylation is incorporated into RNA molecule, thereby leading to an elevated level of CDKN2B - a gene that encodes the protein p15 (a cell growth inhibitor responsible for myeloid differentiation as well as tumour suppression) in their bone marrow [46, 47].

2.14 Acetylcholinesterase inhibitors

Administration of tacrine (a reversible cholinesterase inhibitor) in the treatment of Alzheimer disease, gives rise to an elevated ALT activity in the bloodstream, inferring that there is disruption in the integrity of the hepatocytes. Tacrine's mechanism of liver toxicity may be probably due to the inhibition of cholinesterase activity, resulting in the stimulation of cholinergic coeliac ganglion sensory (or afferent) sympathetic pathway, in which blood constricts, leading to impaired perfusion of the sinusoids and reperfusion injury-mediated by ROS [1].

Despite the basic biochemical indicators discussed above that are associated with drug-induced hepatotoxicity, recent studies have further identified other indicators and these are represented in **Table 1** as shown below:

Drug-induced hepatotoxicity	**Biomarkers of Liver toxicity**	**References**
Acetaminophen (APAP)	Upregulation of mRNA expression of IL-10, IL-36, HO-1, TNFα, MT 1 and 2 and MMP 12 genes.	[48]
D-Galactosamine	Increase in the expressions of NLRP3, NF-kBp65,, IL-6, IL-1β and TNFα genes.	[49]
N-nitrosodiethylamine (NDEA)	Increase MDA level and decrease SOD, CAT, GST, GR, GPx activity.	[50]
Thioacetamide (TAA)	Increase in Anti-PLT Ig level, Increase in the expression of TNFα, HMGB-1 and IL-6 genes. Increase in AST and ALT activity.	[51]
2-Acetylaminofluorene (2-AAF)	Overexpression of iNOS, COX-2, NF-KB, PCNA genes. Increase in xanthine oxidase (XO) activity. Decrease in the activity of SOD, CAT, GST, GR and GPx. Increase in AST and ALT activity. High density of mast cell infiltration.	[52]
Anti-Tuberculosis drugs	Over-expression of NAT2, CYP2E1, ABCB1 genes. Increase in NAD and Bilirubin levels and decrease in HAT activity. Decrease in GST, SOD, CAT activity.	[53]
Anti-retroviral drugs	Increase in ABCB1 gene expression (that is c3435C > T of ABCB1) and CYPs genes (CYP2B6, CYP3A4 and CYP3A5). Increase in IL-1RN, IL-1β, IL-10, HLA-B and C and HLA-DRB1 genes. ALP activity and Total bilirubin (TBil) level increases.	[54, 55]
Anti-hyperlipidemic drugs	Increase in the expression of HLA-DRB1 and SREBP2 genes while CK and HMG-CoA reductase activities increases.	[56]

Abbreviations: *IL (Interleukin), HO 1 (Heme oxygenase 1), TNFα (Alpha tumour nuclear factor), MT (Mitochondrial transition), MMP12 (Mitochondrial membrane permeability 12), NLRP3 (NOD-like receptor protein 3), MDA (Malondialdehyde), iNOS (Inducible nitric oxide synthase), COX 2 (Cyclo-oxygenase 2), NTA2 (N-acetyltransferase 2), HAT (Histone acetyltransferase), CYP (Cytochrome), ABCB1 (ATP binding cassette B1), NAD (Nicotinamide adenine dinucleotide), HLA (Human leucocyte antigen), CK (Creatinine kinase), HMG-CoA (Hydroxylmethylglutaryl Coenzyme A), anti-PLT (anti-platelet), SOD (Superoxide dismutase), CAT (Catalase), GST (Glutathione-S-transferase), GR (Glutathione reductase), GPx (Glutathione peroxidase), ALP (Alkaline phosphatase), HMGB1 (High mobility group box protein 1), SREBP2 (Sterol regulatory element binding protein 2).*

Table 1.
Some recent findings on drug-induced liver toxicity.

3. Conclusions

Drugs primarily serve as therapeutic agents in the treatment and management of various diseases, but over dependent or illicit consumption of drugs, results in hepatotoxicity which confers a detrimental effect on the liver's architecture and functions respectively. Our findings showed that drug-induced hepatotoxicity can cause liver inflammation (associated with excruciating pains), liver transplantation (economically burdensome) as well as death. As a result of these frightening effects outlined above, we hereby conclude that doctor's prescription guideline should be adhered to strictly, indiscriminate use of illicit drugs should be discouraged while regulatory bodies and law enforcement agencies should be empowered to prosecute drug offenders promptly.

Acknowledgement

The expertise of Professor Iheanacho Kizito, Department of Biochemistry, Federal University of Technology, Owerri is well appreciated.

Conflict of interest

The authors declare no conflict of interest in this work.

Author details

Godwin Okwudiri Ihegboro* and Chimaobi James Ononamadu
Department of Biochemistry and Forensic Science, Nigeria Police Academy, Wudil, Kano, Nigeria

*Address all correspondence to: goihegboro@npa.edu.ng

References

[1] Aashish P, Tarun S, Pallavi B. Drug-induced hepatotoxicity: A review. Journal of Applied Pharmaceutical Science. 2012;**2**(5):233-243

[2] William ML. Drug-induced hepatotoxicity. The New England Journal of Medicine. 2003;**349**:474-485. DOI: 10.1056/NEJMra021844

[3] Stefan D, James PH. Drug-induced liver injury. US Gastroenterology & Hepatology Review. 2010;**6**:73-80

[4] Divya S, William CC, Ghanshyam U. Drug-induced liver toxicity and prevention of herbal antioxidants: An overview. Frontiers in Physiology. 2016;**6**:1-18

[5] Chalasani NP, Hayashi PH, Bonkovsky HL, Navarro VJ, Lee WM, Fontana RJ. Practice parameters committee of the American college of gastroenterology. ACG clinical guideline: The diagnosis and management of idiosyncratic drug-induced liver injury. The American Journal of Gastroenterology. 2014;**109**(7):950-966

[6] Donna ML. Drug-induced liver injury: An overview. US Pharmacist. 2016;**41**(12):30-34

[7] Wallace JL. Acetaminophen hepatotoxicity: NO to the rescue. British Journal of Pharmacology. 2004;**143**(1):1-2

[8] Kozer E, Koren G. Management of paracetamol overdose: Current controversies. Drug Safety. 2001;**24**(7):503-512

[9] Qinyu LV, Zhanghul YI. Antipsychotic drugs and liver injury. Shanghai Archives of Psychiatry. 2018;**30**(1):47-51

[10] Diego-Telles-Correia AB, Cortez-Pinto H, Carlos C, Sergio M, et al. Psychotropic drugs and liver disease. A critical review of pharmacokinetics and liver toxicity. World Journal of Gastrointestinal Pharmacology and Therapeutics. 2017;**8**(1):26-38

[11] Apte U. Galactosamine. Encyclopaedia of Toxicology. 3rd ed. Cambridge, USA: Elsevier; 2014. pp. 689-690

[12] Liong EC, Xiao J, Lau TY, Nanji AA, Tipoe GL. Cyclooxygenase inhibitors protect d-galactosamine/lipopolysaccharide induced acute hepatic injury in experimental mice model. Food and Chemical Toxicology. 2012;**50**(3-4):861-866

[13] Wu YH, Hao BJ, Shen E, Meng QL, Hu MH, Zhao Y. Protective properties of *Laggera alata* extract and its principle components against D-Galactosamine injured hepatocytes. Scientia Pharmaceutica. 2012;**80**:447-456

[14] Oliveira MM, Teixeira JC, Vasconcelos-Nóbrega C, Felix LM, Sardão VA, Colaço AA. Mitochondrial and liver oxidative stress alterations induced by N-butyl-N-(4-hydroxybutyl) nitrosamine, relevance for hepatotoxicity. Journal of Applied Toxicology. 2013;**33**(6):434-443

[15] Zhang CL, Zeng T, Zhao ZL, Yu LH, Zhu ZP, Xie KQ. Protective effects of garlic oil on Hepatocarcinomas induced by N-Nitrosodiethylamine in rats. International Journal of Biological Sciences. 2012;**8**(3):363-374

[16] Shaarawy SM, Tohamy AA, Elgendy SM, Elmageed ZY, Bahnasy A, Mohamed MS. Protective effects of garlic

and Silymarin on NDEA-induced rats hepatotoxicity. International Journal of Biological Sciences. 2009;**5**(6):549-557

[17] Tasleem A, Nadeem S. An overview of thioacetamide-induced hepatotoxicity. Toxin Reviews. 2013;**32**(3):43-46

[18] Heather H, Gang H, Yekov K, Diganta S, Weroqi Q, David SM, et al. Metabolism and toxicity of TA and TASO in rats' hepatocytes. Chemical Research in Toxicology. 2012;**25**(9):1955-1963

[19] Ozgun T, Varol S, Mustafa C, Behect I, Adnan A. The protective effects of Silymarin on Thioacetamide-induced liver damage: Measurement of miR-122, miR-192, miR-194 levels. Applied Biochemistry and Biotechnology. 2019;**191**:528-539

[20] Nehal AA, Marwa AI, Mona KG. Hepatoprotective influence of quercetin and Ellagic acid on Thioacetamide-induced hepatotoxicity in rats. Canadian Journal of Physiology and Pharmacology. 2018;**96**(6):624-629

[21] Sebastian M, Artur W, Katarzyna S, Beata W, Waldemar T, Tomasz K, et al. Kynurenic acid protects against Thioacetamide-induced liver injury in rats. Analytical Cellular Pathology. 2018;**1**:1-11

[22] Sehrawat A, Sultana S. Evaluation of possible mechanisms of protective role of *Tamarix gallica* against DEN initiated and 2-AAF promoted hepatocarcinogenesis in male Wistar rats. Life Sciences. 2006;**79**(15):1456-1465

[23] Hermeking H. The miR-34 family in cancer and apoptosis. Cell Death and Differentiation. 2010;**17**(2):193-199

[24] Pogribny IP, Muskhelishvili L, Tryndyak VP, Beland FA. The tumor-promoting activity of 2-acetylaminofluorene is associated with disruption of the p53 signalling pathway and the balance between apoptosis and cell proliferation. Toxicology and Applied Pharmacology. 2009;**235**(3):305-311

[25] Ros JE, Roskams TA, Geuken M, Havinga R, Splinter PL, Petersen BE. ATP binding cassette transporter gene expression in rat liver progenitor cells. Gut. 2003;**52**(7):1060-1067

[26] Iatropoulos MJ, Duanm JD, Jeffreym AM, Leach MW, Hayes AN, Stedman NL. Hepatocellular proliferation and hepatocarcinogen bioactivation in mice with diet induced fatty liver and obesity. Experimental and Toxicologic Pathology. 2012;**65**(4):451-456

[27] Williams GM, Iatropoulos MJ, Jeffrey AM. Thresholds for the effects of 2-Acetylaminofluorene in rat liver. Toxicologic Pathology. 2004;**32** (Suppl. 2):85-91

[28] Rahman S, Sultana S. Protective effects of *Picorrhiza kurroa* extract against 2- acetylaminofluorene-induced hepatotoxicity in Wistar rats. Journal of Environmental Pathology, Toxicology and Oncology. 2007;**26**(3):195-205

[29] Tomioka H, Namba K. Development of anti-tuberculous drugs, current status and future prospects. Kekkaku. 2006;**81**(12):753-774

[30] Tasduq SA, Peerzada K, Koul S, Bhat R, Johri RK. Biochemical manifestations of antituberculosis drugs induced hepatotoxicity and the effect of silymarin. Hepatology Research. 2005;**31**(3):132-135

[31] Saukkonen D, Cohn DL, Jasmer RM, Schenker S, Jereb JA, Nolan CM, et al. An official ATS statement: Hepatotoxicity of anti-tuberculosis therapy. American

Journal of Respiratory and Critical Care Medicine. 2006;**174**:935-952

[32] Yimer G, Ueda N, Habtewold A, Amogne W, Suda A, Riedel KD. Pharmacogenetic & Pharmacokinetic Biomarker for Efavirenz based ARV and rifampicin based anti-TB drug induced liver injury in TB-HIV infected patients. PLoS One. 2011;**6**(12):27810

[33] Roy S, Sannigrahi S, Majumdar S, Ghosh B, Sarkar B. Resveratrol regulates antioxidant status, inhibits cytokine expression and restricts apoptosis in carbon tetrachloride induced rat hepatic injury. Oxidative Medicine and Cellular Longevity. 2011;**2011**:703676

[34] Saraswathy SD, Devi CSS. Antitubercular drugs induced hepatic oxidative stress and ultrastructural changes in rats. BMC Infectious Diseases. 2012;**12**(Suppl. 1):85

[35] Núñez M. Clinical syndromes and consequences of antiretroviral-related hepatotoxicity. Hepatology. 2010;**52**(3):1143-1155

[36] Kovari H, Weber R. Influence of antiretroviral therapy on liver disease. Current Opinion in HIV and AIDS. 2011;**6**(4):272-277

[37] Neuman MG, Schneider M, Nanau RM, Parry C. HIV-antiretroviral therapy induced liver, gastrointestinal, and pancreatic injury. International Journal of Hepatology. 2012;**2012**(2012): 760706

[38] Mendes-Corrêa MC, Andrade HF Jr, Fumica TC, Seixas MI. Hepatic ultrastructural mitochondrial changes prior to antiretroviral therapy in HIV-infected patients in Brazil. Journal of the International Association of Physicians in AIDS Care (Chicago, Ill.). 2008;7(5):252-258

[39] Apostolova N, Gomez-Sucerquia LJ, Moran A, Alvarez A, Blas-Garcia A, Esplugues JV. Enhanced oxidative stress and increased mitochondrial mass during Efavirenz-induced apoptosis in human hepatic cells. British Journal of Pharmacology. 2010;**160**(8):2069-2084

[40] Blas-García A, Apostolova N, Ballesteros D, Monleón D, Morales JM, Rocha M. Inhibition of mitochondrial function by Efavirenz increases lipid content in hepatic cells. Hepatology. 2010;**52**(1):115-125

[41] Burger D, Van der Heiden I, La Porte C, Van der Ende M, Groeneveld P, Richter C. Interpatient variability in the pharmacokinetics of the HIV non-nucleoside reverse transcriptase inhibitor efavirenz, the effect of gender, race, and CYP2B6. Polymorphism. British Journal of Pharmacology. 2006;**61**:148-154

[42] Setzer B, Lebrecht D, Walker UA. Pyrimidine nucleoside depletion sensitizes to the mitochondrial hepatotoxicity of the reverse transcriptase inhibitor stavudine. The American Journal of Pathology. 2008;**172**(3):681-690

[43] Shimizu S, Atsunmi R, Itokawa K, Iwasaki M, Aoki T, Ono C, et al. Metabolism-dependent hepatotoxicity of amodiaquine in glutathione depleted mice. Archives of Toxicology. 2009;**83**:701-707

[44] Manov I, Motanis H, Frumin I, Lancu TC. Hepatotoxicity of anti-inflammatory and analgesic drugs: Ultrastructural aspects. Acta Pharmacologica Sinica. 2006;**27**:259-272

[45] O' Connor N, Dungan PI, Jones AL. Hepatocellular damage from non-steroidal anti-inflammatory drugs. QJM. 2003;**95**(1):787-791

[46] Mohamad MK, Joseph LM. Epigenetic biomarkers in personalized medicine. In: Prognostic Epigenetics. Vol. 15. 2019. pp. 375-395

[47] Shyamala CN. Therapeutics and DNA methylation inhibitors. In: Medical Epigenetics. 2nd ed. Vol. 29. Cambridge, USA: Elsevier; 2021. pp. 937-948

[48] Sina G, Malte B, Itamar G, Amaud H, Andreas W, Jorg K, et al. 3'Mrna sequencing reveals pro-regenerative properties of c5ar1 during resolution of murine acetaminophen-induced liver injury. npj Regenerative Medicine. 2022;**7**:1-10

[49] Yiwei PU, Zhao Cong Y, Xuming MO. Protective effect of Luteolin on D-Galactosamine (D-gal/ Lipopolysacharide (LPS))-induced hepatic injury in mice. BioMed Research International. 2021;**2021**:1-8

[50] Bilat N, Suhail N, Hassan S, Ashrat G, Fatima S, Khan HY, et al. Exacerbation of N-nitrosodiethylamine-induced hepatotoxicity and DNA damage in mice exposed to chronic unpredictable stress. Frontiers in Pharmacology. 2017;**8**:560

[51] Lin YY, Hu CT, Sun DS, et al. Thioacetamide-induced liver damage and thrombocytopenia is associated with induction of anti-platelet autoantibody in mice. Scientific Reports. 2019;**9**:17497

[52] Hassan SK, Khan R, Ali N, Khan AQ, Rehman MU, Tahir M, et al. 18-β-Glycyrrhetinic acid alleviates 2-acetylaminofluorene-induced hepatotoxicity in wistar rats: Role in hyperproliferation, inflammation and oxidative stress. Human & Experimental Toxicology. 2014:1-14

[53] Vidyasagar R, Guruprasad PA. Hepatotoxicity related to anti-tuberculosis drugs: Mechanisms and management. Journal of Clinical and Experimental Hepatology. 2013;**3**:37-49

[54] Andrea G, Agostino R, Felicia SF, Maria LO, Diano C, Stefania C, et al. Clinical and genetic factors associated with increased risk of severe liver toxicity in a monocentric cohort of HIV positive patients receiving nevirapine-based antiretroviral therapy. BMC Infectious Diseases. 2018;**18**:556

[55] Jamie NP, Mohlopheni JM, Nonhlanhla K, Wendy S, Humani N. Mechanistic insights into antiretroviral drug-induced liver injury. Pharmacology Research & Perspectives. 2020;**8**(4):e00598

[56] Natalie CN, Gerald FW, Robert HE. Statin toxicity: Mechanistic insights and clinical implications. Circulation Research. 2019;**124**:328-350

Chapter 2

Oncological-Therapy-Associated Liver Injuries

Victor-Mihai Sacerdoțianu, Costin-Teodor Streba, Ion Rogoveanu, Liliana Streba and Cristin Constantin Vere

Abstract

Drug-induced liver injury (DILI) represents a large group of hepatic disease caused by various treatments, including oncological agents. The liver is an important organ with a role in drug metabolization and excretion and may be affected when oncologic treatment is initiated. The most common liver disease patterns induced by oncologic therapy are steatosis and steatohepatitis, focal nodular hyperplasia, pseudocirrhosis, acute hepatitis, hepatic necrosis, immune-mediated hepatitis, cholestasis, fibrosis and cirrhosis, sinusal obstructive syndrome. In rare cases, chemotherapy treatment is associated with a high-risk hepatic adenoma or hepatocellular carcinoma development. It was demonstrated that the majority of chemotherapy classes can induce these effects on the liver, for example, alkylating agents, antimetabolites, and antitumor antibiotics, but also immunotherapy agents can be involved. The majority of patients that receive oncological treatment who developed liver injury as adverse reactions are identified by symptoms and/or blood test abnormalities. Imaging techniques may be helpful in the diagnosis of oncological-therapy-associated liver injuries, for example, focal nodular hyperplasia, pseudocirrhosis, and sinusal obstructive syndrome. If liver disease occurs as an adverse effect of these agents, the recommendation to stop or continue the administration of oncologic treatment with close monitoring relies upon the risk and benefits of this medication.

Keywords: oncological therapy, immunotherapy, hepatic toxicity, adverse effects, chemotherapy-induced liver injuries

1. Introduction

Drug-induced liver injury (DILI) represents a large group of hepatic diseases caused by various therapeutical agents.

There are two types of DILI, with differences in pharmacologic mechanism and clinical onset patterns. The first type, the predictable one, named *intrinsic* or direct, is typically dose-related and affects a large proportion of exposed individuals if the safe amount is exceeded. It produces distinctive liver lesions, and the onset of clinical and laboratory abnormalities is usually after a short time after drug consumption, hours to days. The effects can be also reproduced using routine animal testing [1].

The second type of DILI, the unpredictable one, named *idiosyncratic*, affects only a small proportion of susceptible individuals exposed to various doses (not dose-related). It produces variable liver injuries, and the onset of clinical and laboratory abnormalities may begin from days to weeks after drug consumption. Usually, the effects cannot be reproduced using routine animal testing [2].

Even the acetaminophen consumption is the cause of the majority of DILI in the USA, in this chapter, our focus will be on injuries induced by oncologic treatment [3]. Despite the chemotherapy possibility of decreasing tumor size and stage, fighting against micrometastatic disease, and prolonging overall survival, it is associated with side effects. The liver is an important organ with a role in drug metabolization and excretion and may be affected when oncologic treatment is initiated.

Several risk factors are associated with a higher incidence of adverse drug reactions, including DILI induced by chemotherapy. Host-related risk factors such as the old age, female sex, HLA class I allele A*33:01, chronic liver disease, and drug-related risk factors such as dose, site of metabolization, and lipophilicity, appear to influence the frequency of occurrence of oncologic treatment hepatic adverse effects. Identifying the risk factors for the development of liver injury after chemotherapy initiation can influence the treatment decision and also improve the patient outcome.

The majority of patients that receive oncological treatment who developed liver injury as adverse reactions are identified by symptoms and/or blood test abnormalities. Elevation of alanine transaminase (ALT), aspartate transaminase (AST), conjugated and total bilirubin (TB), and international normalized ratio (INR) with low values of albumin is frequently revealed in these patients. Symptoms may be absent or nonspecific, or patients can present jaundice, encephalopathy, or coagulopathy manifestation.

DILI, which includes the liver injuries produced by oncological agents, is defined if one of the following criteria is present: (a) more than 5× upper limit of normal ALT value, (b) more than 2× upper limit of normal ALP value (often with the elevation of gamma-glutamyltransferase (GGT)), or (c) more than 3× upper limit of normal ALT value accompanied by more than 2× upper limit of normal TB level value. In practice, there are situations when patients presented with elevated values of the aforementioned blood tests before starting the potential liver harmful treatment, and in this case, the mean of these values replaces the upper limit of normal.

DILI pattern	Hepatocellular injury	Cholestatic injury	Mixed injury
Liver biochemical blood tests abnormalities	≥5× ULN elevation in ALT OR Serum activity ALT to ALP is 5 or more.	≥2× ULN elevation in ALP OR Serum activity ALT to ALP is 2 or less.	serum activity of ALT to ALP is between 2 and 5.
Histological abnormalities	Inflammation, necrosis, and apoptosis; severe necrosis involved zone 3.	Canalicular and hepatocelular cholestasis in zone 3.	more similar changes to that of cholestatic than hepatocellular type.

Table 1.
DILI pattern with his associated biochemical blood tests and histological abnormalities, adapted after EASL clinical practice guidelines, 2019: drug-induced liver injury [2].

The most recent guidelines of EASL (European Association For The Study Of The Liver) classified DILI in "hepatocellular," "cholestatic," or "mixed" types due to the pattern of changes in liver enzymes (**Table 1**) [2].

2. Patterns of oncological-therapy-related liver injury

The most common liver disease patterns induced by oncologic therapy are discussed below, and the agents frequently involved are listed in **Tables 2** and **3**.

2.1 Steatosis and steatohepatitis

NAFLD affects 10–39% of the global population, and only 2% of these patients are caused by drugs. A common effect of chemotherapy is to increase the amount of hepatocellular fat content. Two entities are described, steatosis and steatohepatitis, often known as chemotherapy-induced acute steatohepatitis, "CASH." Steatosis is defined by the accumulation of lipids within hepatocytes without inflammatory foci. Steatohepatitis is the lipid accumulation with concurrent inflammation of liver parenchyma on hepatocytes that appear enlarged (ballooning phenomes) and can lead to degeneration [4–6].

Class	Drug name	Patterns of drug-associated liver adverse effects
Alkylating agents	Cyclophosphamide	sinusoidal obstructive syndrome; cholestasis; acute hepatitis; hepatic necrosis;
	Chlorambucil	cholestasis; sinusoidal obstructive syndrome;
	Oxaliplatin	sinusoidal obstructive syndrome; pseudocirrhosis; steatosis; focal nodular hyperplasia;
	Ifosfamide	acute hepatitis;
	Melphalan	sinusoidal obstructive syndrome; acute hepatitis;
	Busulfan	sinusoidal obstructive syndrome; acute hepatitis; cholestasis;
Anti-metabolites	5-Fluorouracil	pseudocirrhosis; steatosis; acute hepatitis; sinusoidal obstructive syndrome; cholestasis;
	Methotrexate	hepatic necrosis; steatosis; steatohepatitis; focal nodular hyperplasia; acute hepatitis; fibrosis and cirrhosis;
	6-mercaptopurine	sinusoidal obstructive syndrome; cholestasis; focal nodular hyperplasia; acute hepatitis;
	6-thioguanine	sinusoidal obstructive syndrome; focal nodular hyperplasia; peliosis hepatitis; fibrosis;
	Capecitabine	acute hepatitis;
	Gemcitabine	pseudocirrhosis; acute hepatitis; cholestasis;
	Cytarabine	cholestasis; sinusoidal obstructive syndrome;
	Floxuridine	acute hepatitis; cholestasis; steatosis;
	Azathioprine	cholestasis; sinusoidal obstructive syndrome;
Antitumor antibiotics	Doxorubicin	acute hepatitis; cholestasis; sinusoidal obstructive syndrome;
	Dacarbazine	sinusoidal obstructive syndrome; hepatic necrosis;
	Dactinomycin	sinusoidal obstructive syndrome; steatosis;

Class	Drug name	Patterns of drug-associated liver adverse effects
	Mitomycin C	sinusoidal obstructive syndrome; acute hepatitis; steatosis;
	Actinomycin	acute hepatitis; sinusoidal obstructive syndrome;
	Bleomycin	acute hepatitis; steatosis;
	Mithramycin	hepatic necrosis;
Isomerase inhibitors	Etoposide	hepatic necrosis; acute hepatitis; cholestasis;
	Irinotecan	steatosis; steatohepatitis; sinusoidal obstructive syndrome;
	Topotecan	cholestasis;
Taxanes	Paclitaxel	cholestasis; sinusoidal obstructive syndrome;
	Docetaxel	cholestasis;
Hormone therapy	Tamoxifen	steatosis; steatohepatitis; cholestasis;
	Anastrozole	steatosis; acute hepatitis;
	Estrogens	cholestasis; hepatic adenoma and hepatocellular carcinoma; peliosis hepatis; sinusoidal obstructive syndrome;
Vinca alkaloids	Vincristine	sinusoidal obstructive syndrome; acute hepatitis;
	Vinorelbine	cholestasis;
	Vinblastine	acute hepatitis;
Platinum agents	Cisplatine	acute hepatitis; steatosis; sinusoidal obstructive syndrome; cholestasis;
	Carboplatin	sinusoidal obstructive syndrome;
Nitrosoureas	Carmustine	acute hepatitis; sinusoidal obstructive syndrome;
	Lomustine	acute hepatitis;

Table 2.
Commonly used agents in chemotherapy and their associated liver-related side effects.

Various therapeutic agents used in oncology can induce steatosis or steatohepatitis. Regimens that contain antitumoral molecules such as 5-fluorouracil, methotrexate, tamoxifen, irinotecan, L-asparaginase, oxaliplatin, mitomycin C, bleomycin sulfate, and dactinomycin were linked with fatty liver transformation [7, 8]. Usually, specific changes are detected after a period of 3–12 months of chemotherapy.

Treatments recommended for patients diagnosed with cancer contain not only antitumoral agents. Associated medication used in oncology can also induce nonalcoholic fatty liver disease. Glucocorticoids used for induction treatment of acute leukemia may cause macrovesicular steatosis [9].

A high number, up to 85%, of patients treated with regimens mentioned above develop CASH due to altered lipoprotein synthesis and therefore abnormal lipid metabolism. The development of steatohepatitis is based on an abnormal function of hepatocyte mitochondria and peroxisomes, inside which the process of oxidation of fatty acids (FAO) takes place. Several chemotherapy agents inhibit free fatty acids (FFA) β-oxidation, which promotes the accumulation of reactive oxygen species (ROS) and lipid peroxidation and increases oxidative stress in hepatocytes. All these processes lead to CASH. At the same time, lipid peroxidation stimulates stellate cell activation, fibrosis, and necrosis of hepatocytes.

Class	Drug name	Patterns of drug-associated liver adverse effects
Tyrosine kinase inhibitors	Imatinib	acute hepatitis;
	Erlotinib	cholestasis;
	Lapatinib	acute hepatitis;
	Gefitinib	acute hepatitis;
	Pazopanib	hepatic necrosis;
	Sorafenib	acute hepatitis; cholestasis;
	Regorafenib	hepatic necrosis;
	Sunitinib	hepatic necrosis;
	Bortezomib	acute hepatitis;
	Idelalisib	acute hepatitis;
Monoclonal antibodies	Trastuzumab	acute hepatitis; nodular regenerative hyperplasia;
	Ipilimumab	immune-mediated hepatitis;
	Durvalumab	immune-mediated hepatitis;
	Nivolumab	immune-mediated hepatitis;
	Cetuximab	steatosis;
	Pembrolizumab	immune-mediated hepatitis;
	Atezolizumab	immune-mediated hepatitis;
	Gemtuzumab	sinusoidal obstructive syndrome;
	Rituximab	acute hepatitis;
	Bretuximab vedotin	hepatic necrosis;
	Avelumab	immune-mediated hepatitis;
Immunomodulatory drugs	Lenalidomide	cholestasis;
	Pegylated interferon α	immune-mediated hepatitis;
	Interleukin2	cholestasis; acute hepatitis; sinusoidal obstructive syndrome;
Biological agents	L-Asparaginase	hepatic necrosis; steatosis;

Table 3.
Immunomodulatory agents in chemotherapy and their associated liver-related side effects.

The intramitochondrial accumulation of tamoxifen leads to the inhibition of FFA β-oxidation, ATP synthesis, and cellular respiration. Another mechanism of steatosis and steatohepatitis is explained by the alteration of lysosomal phospholipid metabolism, which promotes the activation of the adenosine pathway and therefore increases FFA synthesis and also coenzyme A sequestration. This mechanism was observed in patients undergoing treatment with irinotecan and methotrexate. For methotrexate, the increased level of homocysteine due to impaired methylenetetrahydrofolate reductase leads to increased pro-inflammatory cytokines and hepatic stellate cell activation, which promote liver fibrosis. Increased expression of acyl-coenzyme A oxidase 1 (ACOX1) was observed for patients treated with 5-fluorouracil and irinotecan. Inhibition of mitochondrial FFA β -oxidation and reduced expression of carnitine palmitoyl-transferase and ACOX1 induction were observed for irinotecan [10].

ACOX1 is the first limiting enzyme of peroxisomal FAO and may be increased as a response to decreased mitochondrial FFA β-oxidation. A high level of ACOX1 leads to increased expression of pro-inflammatory genes and a high amount of ROS, processes associated with immune cell infiltration. A hepatic steatosis liver can progress to steatohepatitis if contained hepatocytes own altered mitochondrial FFA β-oxidation and high amounts of ROS and inflammation. Mitochondria can be a direct target of every chemotherapy agent via cytotoxicity effect, and every agent can also have multiple pathways to induce steatosis or steatohepatitis [11].

Histologically, there are no marked differences between metabolic steatohepatitis and CASH. Even actually is rare recommended, if liver biopsy is performed on this patient, microvesicular steatosis is usually described. Distribution can be focal, multifocal, or diffuse. Macroscopic, fatty liver has a yellowish appearance and may be enlarged.

Recognition of this liver disease is important for adequate management that improves the prognosis. Usually, clinical manifestations of patients with chemotherapy-induced steatosis and steatohepatitis are subtle. Transaminase levels show elevation of ALT/AST. Steatosis and steatohepatitis liver is characterized by hyperechogenicity with posterior beam attenuation on transabdominal ultrasound examination. On computed tomography, a reduction in liver parenchymal attenuation can be observed when compared with the spleen. With high accuracy, magnetic resonance imaging can quantify the number of lipids in the liver due to spectroscopy and elastography available modes. A reduction in liver signal intensity is described in out-of-phase imaging for patients with steatohepatitis [12–14]. Delayed regeneration and prolonged liver disfunction were observed in oncologic patients with steatosis and more obvious with steatohepatitis, which was associated with a higher risk of postoperative hepatic failure, infections, and longer period of the intensive-care-unit stay [4, 15]. Repeated chemotherapy cycles are responsible for more severe inflammation, fact that worsens hepatocellular damage and leads to the development of fibrosis, cirrhosis, and liver failure [16, 17]. A limited CASH risk with the best oncologic treatment effects was observed for chemotherapy regimens with a maximum duration of 4 months [18].

For patients diagnosed with cancer, blood lipid and transaminase levels should be performed before initiation and regularly during oncologic treatment. Steatosis and steatohepatitis are in most cases reversible even though they can persist for a few weeks or months after treatment completion [7, 19]. Once the diagnosis was confirmed, the recommendation to stop or continue the administration of oncologic agents with close monitoring relies upon the risk and benefits of this medication. Healthy eating habits and limited high-fat alimentation are recommended to prevent increased blood lipid levels and worsening steatosis or steatohepatitis. Hepatoprotective drug administration, to prevent the worsening damage to the liver, is indicated [20].

Risk factors for CASH occurrence can be patient-related (metabolic syndromes, obesity, diabetes, dyslipidemia, alcohol abuse, preexisting chronic liver disease or hepatic location of the tumor, genetic polymorphism, gut microbiota, and chemotherapy history) or drug-related (cumulative or maximum dose of treatment or combination of more agents) [4]. Special attention is required for women with breast cancer with the A2 allele of CYP17A1 due to the associated increased risk of developing steatosis when treated with tamoxifen [21, 22].

2.2 Focal nodular hyperplasia

Focal nodular hyperplasia is the second most common benign hepatic lesion with unclear pathogenesis. Some explanations for this lesion may include a similar mechanism to focal sinusoidal obstruction syndrome [23].

Some agents used in oncology such as 6-thioguanine and oxaliplatin have an increased risk of inducing nodular hyperplasia and early fibrosis [24, 25]. Focal nodular hyperplasia is characterized by solitary or multiple lesions in liver parenchyma, which usually appear on CT as homogeneous, isodense, or mildly hypodense images. Contrast-enhanced CT shows arterial hyperenhancement, and late enhancement can be seen when a central scar is visible. These lesions may be incorrectly labeled as hypervascular liver metastasis. Characteristic MRI features for focal nodular hyperplasia are nonspherical shape lesions with imprecise margins and particularly hyperenhanced zones in the hepatobiliary phase for specific contrast agents. Signal isointensity on T1- and T2-weighted images, the absence of halo enhancement, and the absence of restriction to water diffusion in the echo-planar sequence are other characteristics that support the diagnosis of focal nodular hyperplasia [23, 26].

2.3 Pseudocirrhosis

Pseudocirrhosis is an imagistic term characterized by hepatic nodularity due to diffuse regenerative nodular hyperplasia but with insignificant fibrosis, different from the classic histopathological attributes of cirrhosis, features that appear after oncologic treatment initiation [27]. Pseudocirrhosis is associated with antineoplastic drugs used for the treatment of metastatic breast, colon, and pancreatic cancers. These agents are oxaliplatin, 5-fluorouracil, gemcitabine, capecitabine, irinotecan, methotrexate, and tamoxifen [28]. It can also appear in patients with carcinoid tumors and Hodgkin lymphoma.

Pseudocirrhosis can represent a cause of portal hypertension and even liver failure, but it lacks the typical clinical and paraclinical features of cirrhosis. The synthetic function of the liver is usually preserved.

On CT examination, pseudocirrhosis looks like macronodular cirrhosis with capsular retraction, diffuse nodularity, lower liver volume, and hypertrophy of the caudate lobe. For up to 9% of cases, signs of portal hypertension, including portosystemic shunts, can appear on imaging evaluation. The severe capsular retraction has been described in some cases of liver metastasis from breast cancer, and those must be excluded due to different treatments and prognoses that are associated with this stage [6, 23].

2.4 Acute hepatitis

Multiple oncological agents are involved in acute hepatitis occurrence, with high-frequency vinblastine, rituximab, etoposide, anastrozole, 6-mercaptopurine, 5-fluorouracil, lapatinib [6, 29, 30]. Even though not routinely indicated, if liver biopsy is performed on patients that underwent treatment with anastrozole, the histopathology report revealed necrosis of hepatocytes limited in acinar zone 3. This zone is related to P450 isoenzymes that are involved in drug metabolism. Histopathological report of liver biopsy of patients treated with lapatinib revealed portal-to-portal and portal-to-central bridging necrosis and hepatocellular necrosis in acinar zone 1 [31, 32]. Etoposide-induced acute hepatitis is described as a viral hepatitis pattern [29].

Clinical manifestation of acute hepatitis can range from mild symptoms to ill-appearing patients. Usually, AST and ALT are markedly increased. Imaging findings are nonspecific and may include hepatomegaly with decreased attenuation, splenomegaly, wall thickening of gallbladder, ascites, and periportal edema. Severe forms of acute hepatitis appear in patients with prior chronic hepatitis B or C due to reactivation when treated with rituximab. Patients with MHC class II alleles HLA-DQA1∗02:01, DQB1∗02:02, or DRB1∗07:01 are at high risk of liver injury if receiving regimens with lapatinib [6, 33].

Acute hepatitis induced by anticancer treatment rapidly improved after drug withdrawal. Liver enzymes and bilirubin return to normal values after a few months of treatment discontinuation [5].

2.5 Hepatic necrosis

Acute liver failure due to hepatic necrosis is a major and worrisome complication of chemotherapy-induced liver injury. Oncologic agents that produce acute hepatitis are more likely to cause hepatic necrosis. Mithramycin, etoposide, and dacarbazine are some of these offending drugs. Mithramycin also known as plicamycin is an antineoplastic antibiotic that has been reported as the most hepatotoxic chemotherapeutic drug capable of causing liver necrosis. Histopathologic reports of the hepatic biopsy reveal centrilobular necrosis.

Clinically, patients with hepatic necrosis develop acute encephalopathy with deterioration of liver synthetic function. Almost all patients receiving plicamycin have increased levels of LDH, aminotransferases, and alkaline phosphatase with normal values of bilirubin. These modifications occur on the first day of treatment, reach the maximum level the next day, and then decrease to normal 3 weeks after treatment cessation. When severe necrosis develops, a computer tomography scan reveals a substantial decrease in the enhancement of liver parenchyma and cystic appearance [6, 34, 35].

2.6 Immune-mediated hepatitis

Metastatic melanoma, non-small-cell lung cancer hepatocellular carcinoma, and urothelial carcinoma are types of cancer that benefit from immunotherapy agents' efficacy. Side effects are not rare for this class of treatment and are named immune-related adverse effects, including the liver with immune-mediated hepatitis [36].

Immune checkpoints are cytotoxic T-lymphocyte antigen 4 (CTLA-4), programmed cell death 1 (PD-1), and programmed cell death ligand 1 (PD-L1). Monoclonal antibodies against these targets are ipilimumab against CTLA-4, pembrolizumab, nivolumab against PD-1 and atezolizumab, avelumab, and durvalumab against PD-L1. From this list, the higher hepatotoxicity was found for CTLA-4 inhibitors, ipilimumab. Patients diagnosed with metastatic melanoma develop immune-mediated hepatitis in 2–9% of cases if they are treated with ipilimumab, and if dacarbazine is associated, the percentage rises up to 31.6% [37, 38].

Immunotherapy contains agents that increase the host's immune system to fight against tumors, but the subsequent uncontrolled T cell activation is responsible for hepatotoxicity and liver disease. Liver biopsy revealed diffuse T-cell infiltrate, eosinophil infiltration, portal, and periportal inflammation, and spotty or confluent necrosis [39–41]. Usually, patients are asymptomatic and, in rare cases, fevers, malaise, or symptoms related to fulminant liver failure can be present. Elevation in serum of ALT, AST, and bilirubin occurs especially after ipilimumab. Anti-nuclear, anti-smooth muscle, or other autoimmune hepatitis antibodies are negative. These clinical and paraclinical abnormalities occur from 6 to 14 weeks after immunotherapy initiation or after three doses of this regimen [42, 43]. Some risk factors contribute to a higher chance of liver injury development: a higher dose of treatment, multiple agents association, preexisting liver disease, or autoimmune diathesis [44].

Treatment with corticosteroids or mycophenolate mofetil is indicated for patients with important hepatotoxicity after immunotherapy for cancer [39]. HLA-DRB1*07:01 allele is associated with an increased risk for lapatinib liver injury. Infliximab should not be indicated due to the risk of hepatotoxicity [45, 46].

2.7 Cholestasis

Chemotherapeutic regimens include kinase inhibitors (e.g., erlotinib, sorafenib, nilotinib), thiopurines (6-mercaptopurine and azathioprine), estrogens, 5-fluorouracil, cytarabine, interleukin-2, alkylating agents (chlorambucil, cyclophosphamide, cisplatin), and mitomycin are associated with cholestatic liver injury [29, 35].

Thiopurines cause a variety of DILI phenotypes that can be intrinsic or idiosyncratic with a mixed or cholestatic form of hepatic injury [47]. Intrahepatic cholestasis is the most frequent type of injury in patients undergoing treatment with 6-mercaptopurine (frequently when the daily dose exceeds 2 mg/kg). Azathioprine may produce hepatic injury, but less frequently than 6-mercaptopurine, and this one has been related to a mild form of liver toxicity; however, long-term use can cause cholestatic liver disease [35].

Significant hepatotoxicity has been linked to fluorodeoxyuridine, a metabolite of fluorouracil that was previously administered through the hepatic artery to patients with hepatic metastases from colorectal cancer. In several cases, the treatment has been linked to irreversible intrahepatic and extrahepatic biliary strictures. Monitoring of aminotransferases helps with identifying the right time for drug discontinuation when the liver is suffering [29].

Interleukin-2 therapy is used in melanoma and renal cell cancers, and a lot of patients undergoing this treatment can develop a deep and reversible intrahepatic cholestasis with increased serum levels of biochemical markers of cholestasis. Some potential physiopathological mechanisms may include chemical hepatitis and biliary sclerosis. Allopurinol can block xanthine oxidase involved in drug metabolism, which rises hepatotoxicity. Histologically features of this hepatic injury appear as cholestasis with variable hepatocellular necrosis. Laboratory tests show elevated levels of bilirubin, alkaline phosphatase, and aminotransferases. Jaundice is the clinical feature that is associated with this type of hepatotoxicity [6]. In conclusion, cholestasis is induced by a multitude of antineoplastic drugs and withdrawal usually leads to recovery of the liver and jaundice disappearance [29].

2.8 Fibrosis and cirrhosis

Liver fibrosis and cirrhosis induced by chemotherapy are usually associated with alkylating agents, 6-thioguanine, and methotrexate.

Methotrexate is a folic acid antagonist that inhibits the proliferation of certain body cells, particularly those that are multiplying rapidly such as tumor cells, bone marrow cells, and skin cells. Long-term methotrexate treatment, commonly used to treat severe psoriasis or rheumatoid arthritis, can induce hepatic fibrosis, which leads to cirrhosis without producing significant symptoms [48]. The use of methotrexate as maintenance therapy in children with acute leukemia was related to fibrosis and cirrhosis development in multiple cases [49, 50]. Furthermore, cirrhosis induced by methotrexate has led to the transplantation of the liver in an important number of patients. Hepatic stellate cells have a central role in the physiopathological mechanism. The hepatic test may be normal or ALT can be temporarily increased. In rare cases, a liver biopsy may be necessary to confirm the diagnosis [29].

Patients who receive treatment with methotrexate need rigorous monitoring, especially those who have both obesity and diabetes [51]. It has been demonstrated that folic acid may reduce hepatic injury [29].

2.9 Sinusal obstructive syndrome

Previously named veno-occlusive disease, sinusoidal obstruction syndrome is the last step of hepatic sinusoidal injury evolution. The most exposed are patients who receive cytoreductive chemotherapy combined with radiotherapy or are in the setting of bone marrow transplantation [52].

Cyclophosphamide, oxaliplatin, irinotecan, 5-fluorouracil, 6-mercaptopurine, dacarbazine, vincristine, mitomycin-C, cytarabine, busulfan are chemotherapy agents involved in hepatic sinusoidal injury [53–58]. Usually, sinusoidal obstruction syndrome occurs 5 weeks or later after administration of the aforementioned agents [23].

Direct injury of endothelial cells that lined the hepatic sinusoids is the mechanism of this type of disease. Endothelial injury promotes erythrocyte extravasation and aggregation into space of Disse, which impairs venous outflow. This leads to sinusoidal congestion. The next step is a fibrotic reaction due to hepatic stellate cell activation, which leads to presinusoidal collagen deposit and central venules obstruction with sinusoidal obstruction syndrome development and centrilobular necrosis. Increased activity of matrix metalloproteinase 2 and 9 may facilitate this process [59, 60].

No direct hepatocellular function alteration was observed for this entity [61, 62]. Histological findings vary from hepatic sinusoidal dilatation to subendothelial fibrin deposits associated with centrilobular necrosis of hepatocytes and low grades of nodular regenerative changes. The macroscopic liver had a bluish marbled appearance. Due to the area affected, sinusoidal obstruction syndrome can be classified into mild, moderate, or severe if less than 1/3, 1/3–2/3, or more than 2/3 of the lobule was affected [7, 63]. There are three phases of sinusoidal obstruction syndrome: acute, subacute, and chronic. Patients may present painful hepatomegaly, short periods of jaundice, weight gain, and encephalopathy. Some patients have splenomegaly and ascites due to portal hypertension. Transient elevation of transaminases and bilirubin can be revealed on blood tests [64, 65].

Transabdominal ultrasound revealed hepatosplenomegaly, decreased flow in portal vein on Doppler mode, ascites, and gallbladder wall thickening. In the hepatobiliary phase of gadoxetic-acid-enhanced MRI, sinusoidal obstruction syndrome can present a diffuse heterogenous reticular pattern. CT and MRI findings also include narrowing of main hepatic veins [66, 67].

Viral hepatitis, Budd-Chiari syndrome, or other forms of DILI must be excluded before sinusoidal obstruction syndrome diagnosis. The evolution of persistent sinusoidal obstruction syndrome is represented by progression to regenerative nodular hyperplasia followed by fibrosis and cirrhosis development. Also, sinusoidal obstruction syndrome can impair chemotherapy response and liver regeneration after resection, which worsens prognosis. Patients with hepatitis C infection, stem cell transplant recipients, and those treated for Hodgkin lymphoma are more susceptible to developing sinusoidal obstruction syndrome after specific chemotherapeutic regimens. In addition, patients with colorectal cancer with hepatic metastasis are more susceptible to sinusoidal obstruction syndrome development if the oxaliplatin or irinotecan treatment is combined with 5-fluorouracil [57, 58, 68].

Sinusoidal obstruction syndrome changes can be reversible after cessation of chemotherapy. Supportive therapy and administration of bevacizumab or defibrotide sodium can reduce liver injury and may improve the efficacy of systemic treatment. Delaying surgery for patients with suspected sinusoidal obstruction syndrome can be an option [69].

Except for the patterns discussed above, other chemotherapy-induced liver disease exists, with a low frequency. For example, estrogens, which are used for advanced prostate cancer, are associated with a high risk of peliosis hepatitis, hepatic adenoma, or hepatocellular carcinoma development [70].

Despite the pattern of liver disease induced by oncologic agents administration, a correct diagnosis and management may reduce the hepatic damage and improve the prognosis of these patients.

Acknowledgements

This work was supported by a grant of the Romanian Ministry of Education and Research, CNCS—UEFISCDI, project number PN-III-P1-1.1-TE-2019-1474, within PNCDI III.

Author details

Victor-Mihai Sacerdoţianu[1], Costin-Teodor Streba[1,2*], Ion Rogoveanu[1], Liliana Streba[3] and Cristin Constantin Vere[1]

1 Department of Gastroenterology, University of Medicine and Pharmacy of Craiova, Romania

2 Department of Pulmonology, University of Medicine and Pharmacy of Craiova, Romania

3 Department of Oncology, University of Medicine and Pharmacy of Craiova, Romania

*Address all correspondence to: costinstreba@gmail.com

References

[1] Roth RA, Ganey PE. Intrinsic versus idiosyncratic drug-induced hepatotoxicity—Two villains or one? The Journal of Pharmacology and Experimental Therapeutics. 2010;**332**(3):692-697. DOI: 10.1124/jpet.109.162651

[2] Andrade RJ, Aithal GP, Björnsson ES, Kaplowitz N, Kullak-Ublick GA, Larrey D, et al. EASL clinical practice guidelines: Drug-induced liver injury. Journal of Hepatology. 2019;**70**(6):1222-1261. DOI: 10.1016/j.jhep.2019.02.014

[3] Kaplowitz N. Acetaminophen hepatoxicity: What do we know, what don't we know, and what do we do next? Hepatology. 2004;**40**(1):23-26. DOI: 10.1002/hep.20312

[4] Meunier L, Larrey D. Chemotherapy-associated steatohepatitis. Annals of Hepatology. 2020;**19**(6):597-601. DOI: 10.1016/j.aohep.2019.11.012

[5] Maor Y, Malnick S. Liver injury induced by anticancer chemotherapy and radiation therapy. International Journal of Hepatology. 2013;**2013**:815105. DOI: 10.1155/2013/815105

[6] Sharma A, Houshyar R, Bhosale P, Choi JI, Gulati R, Lall C. Chemotherapy induced liver abnormalities: An imaging perspective. Clinical and Molecular Hepatology. 2014;**20**(3):317-326. DOI: 10.3350/cmh.2014.20.3.317

[7] Vigano L, De Rosa G, Toso C, Andres A, Ferrero A, Roth A, et al. Reversibility of chemotherapy-related liver injury. Journal of Hepatology. 2017;**67**(1):84-91. DOI: 10.1016/j.jhep.2017.02.031

[8] Zhao J, van Mierlo KMC, Gómez-Ramírez J, Kim H, Pilgrim CHC, Pessaux P, et al. Systematic review of the influence of chemotherapy-associated liver injury on outcome after partial hepatectomy for colorectal liver metastases. The British Journal of Surgery. 2017;**104**(8):990-1002. DOI: 10.1002/bjs.10572

[9] Rieder H, Meyer zum Büschenfelde KH, Ramadori G. Functional spectrum of sinusoidal endothelial liver cells. Filtration, endocytosis, synthetic capacities and intercellular communication. Journal of Hepatology. 1992;**15**(1-2):237-250. DOI: 10.1016/0168-8278(92)90042-n

[10] Mahli A, Saugspier M, Koch A, Sommer J, Dietrich P, Lee S, et al. ERK activation and autophagy impairment are central mediators of irinotecan-induced steatohepatitis. Gut. 2018;**67**(4):746-756. DOI: 10.1136/gutjnl-2016-312485

[11] Labbe G, Pessayre D, Fromenty B. Drug-induced liver injury through mitochondrial dysfunction: Mechanisms and detection during preclinical safety studies. Fundamental & Clinical Pharmacology. 2008;**22**(4):335-353. DOI: 10.1111/j.1472-8206.2008.00608.x

[12] McGettigan MJ, Menias CO, Gao ZJ, Mellnick VM, Hara AK. Imaging of drug-induced complications in the gastrointestinal system. Radiographics. 2016;**36**(1):71-87. DOI: 10.1148/rg.2016150132

[13] Guglielmo FF, Venkatesh SK, Mitchell DG. Liver MR elastography technique and image interpretation: Pearls and pitfalls. Radiographics. 2019;**39**(7):1983-2002. DOI: 10.1148/rg.2019190034

[14] Salameh N, Larrat B, Abarca-Quinones J, Pallu S, Dorvillius M, Leclercq I, et al. Early detection of steatohepatitis in fatty rat liver by using MR elastography. Radiology. 2009;**253**(1):90-97. DOI: 10.1148/radiol.2523081817

[15] McCormack L, Petrowsky H, Jochum W, Furrer K, Clavien PA. Hepatic steatosis is a risk factor for postoperative complications after major hepatectomy: A matched case-control study. Annals of Surgery. 2007;**245**(6):923-930. DOI: 10.1097/01.sla.0000251747.80025.b7

[16] Mulhall BP, Ong JP, Younossi ZM. Non-alcoholic fatty liver disease: An overview. Journal of Gastroenterology and Hepatology. 2002;**17**(11):1136-1143. DOI: 10.1046/j.1440-1746.2002.02881.x

[17] Ong JP, Younossi ZM. Epidemiology and natural history of NAFLD and NASH. Clinics in Liver Disease. 2007;**11**(1):1-16, vii. DOI: 10.1016/j.cld.2007.02.009

[18] White RR, Schwartz LH, Munoz JA, Raggio G, Jarnagin WR, Fong Y, et al. Assessing the optimal duration of chemotherapy in patients with colorectal liver metastases. Journal of Surgical Oncology. 2008;**97**(7):601-604. DOI: 10.1002/jso.21042

[19] Torrisi JM, Schwartz LH, Gollub MJ, Ginsberg MS, Bosl GJ, Hricak H. CT findings of chemotherapy-induced toxicity: What radiologists need to know about the clinical and radiologic manifestations of chemotherapy toxicity. Radiology. 2011;**258**(1):41-56. DOI: 10.1148/radiol.10092129

[20] Sun Y, Zhang N, Ding Y-L, Yu L-J, Cai J, Ma D, et al. Effect of lipid metabolism disorder on liver function in patients with malignant tumors after chemotherapy: A case-control study. Lipids in Health and Disease. 2019;**18**(1):108. DOI: 10.1186/s12944-019-1063-y

[21] Schumacher JD, Guo GL. Mechanistic review of drug-induced steatohepatitis. Toxicology and Applied Pharmacology. 2015;**289**(1):40-47. DOI: 10.1016/j.taap.2015.08.022

[22] Alexander JL, Wilson ID, Teare J, Marchesi JR, Nicholson JK, Kinross JM. Gut microbiota modulation of chemotherapy efficacy and toxicity. Nature Reviews. Gastroenterology & Hepatology. 2017;**14**(6):356-365. DOI: 10.1038/nrgastro.2017.20

[23] Torri GB, Soldatelli MD, Luersen GF, Ghezzi CLA. Imaging of chemotherapy-induced liver toxicity: An illustrated overview. Hepatic. Oncology. 2021;**8**(4):HEP32. DOI: 10.2217/hep-2020-0026

[24] Geller SA, Dubinsky MC, Poordad FF, Vasiliauskas EA, Cohen AH, Abreu MT, et al. Early hepatic nodular hyperplasia and submicroscopic fibrosis associated with 6-thioguanine therapy in inflammatory bowel disease. The American Journal of Surgical Pathology. 2004;**28**(9):1204-1211. DOI: 10.1097/01.pas.0000128665.12063.97

[25] Satti MB, Weinbren K, Gordon-Smith EC. 6-thioguanine as a cause of toxic veno-occlusive disease of the liver. Journal of Clinical Pathology. 1982;**35**(10):1086-1091. DOI: 10.1136/jcp.35.10.1086

[26] Han NY, Park BJ, Sung DJ, Kim MJ, Cho SB, Lee CH, et al. Chemotherapy-induced focal hepatopathy in patients with gastrointestinal malignancy: gadoxetic acid-enhanced and diffusion-weighted MR imaging with clinical-pathologic correlation. Radiology. 2014;**271**(2):416-425. DOI: 10.1148/radiol.13131810

[27] Jeong WK, Choi SY, Kim J. Pseudocirrhosis as a complication after chemotherapy for hepatic metastasis from breast cancer. Clinical and Molecular Hepatology. 2013;**19**(2):190-194. DOI: 10.3350/cmh.2013.19.2.190

[28] Kang SP, Taddei T, McLennan B, Lacy J. Pseudocirrhosis in a pancreatic cancer patient with liver metastases: A case report of complete resolution of pseudocirrhosis with an early recognition and management. World Journal of Gastroenterology. 2008;**14**(10):1622-1624. DOI: 10.3748/wjg.14.1622

[29] Ricart AD. Drug-induced liver injury in oncology. Annals of Oncology. 2017;**28**(8):2013-2020. DOI: 10.1093/annonc/mdx158

[30] Grigorian A, O'Brien CB. Hepatotoxicity secondary to chemotherapy. Journal of Clinical and Translational Hepatology. 2014;**2**(2):95-102. DOI: 10.14218/JCTH.2014.00011

[31] Inno A, Basso M, Vecchio FM, Marsico VA, Cerchiaro E, D'Argento E, et al. Anastrozole-related acute hepatitis with autoimmune features: A case report. BMC Gastroenterology. 2011;**11**:32. DOI: 10.1186/1471-230x-11-32

[32] Peroukides S, Makatsoris T, Koutras A, Tsamandas A, Onyenadum A, Labropoulou-Karatza C, et al. Lapatinib-induced hepatitis: A case report. World Journal of Gastroenterology. 2011;**17**(18):2349-2352. DOI: 10.3748/wjg.v17.i18.2349

[33] Faggioli P, De Paschale M, Tocci A, Luoni M, Fava S, De Paoli A, et al. Acute hepatic toxicity during cyclic chemotherapy in non Hodgkin's lymphoma. Haematologica. 1997;**82**(1):38-42

[34] Kennedy BJ. Metabolic and toxic effects of mithramycin during tumor therapy. The American Journal of Medicine. 1970;**49**(4):494-503. DOI: 10.1016/s0002-9343(70)80044-4

[35] King PD, Perry MC. Hepatotoxicity of chemotherapy. The Oncologist. 2001;**6**(2):162-176. DOI: 10.1634/theoncologist.6-2-162

[36] Brown ZJ, Heinrich B, Steinberg SM, Yu SJ, Greten TF. Safety in treatment of hepatocellular carcinoma with immune checkpoint inhibitors as compared to melanoma and non-small cell lung cancer. Journal for Immunotherapy of Cancer. 2017;**5**(1):93. DOI: 10.1186/s40425-017-0298-2

[37] Kaplowitz N. Avoiding idiosyncratic DILI: Two is better than one. Hepatology. 2013;**58**(1):15-17. DOI: 10.1002/hep.26295

[38] McEuen K, Borlak J, Tong W, Chen M. Associations of drug lipophilicity and extent of metabolism with drug-induced liver injury. International Journal of Molecular Sciences. 2017;**18**(7):1335. DOI: 10.3390/ijms18071335

[39] Weber JS, Kähler KC, Hauschild A. Management of immune-related adverse events and kinetics of response with ipilimumab. Journal of Clinical Oncology. 2012;**30**(21):2691-2697. DOI: 10.1200/jco.2012.41.6750

[40] Kleiner DE, Berman D. Pathologic changes in ipilimumab-related hepatitis in patients with metastatic melanoma. Digestive Diseases and Sciences. 2012;**57**(8):2233-2240. DOI: 10.1007/s10620-012-2140-5

[41] Johncilla M, Misdraji J, Pratt DS, Agoston AT, Lauwers GY, Srivastava A, et al. Ipilimumab-associated hepatitis: Clinicopathologic characterization in a series of 11 cases. The American Journal of Surgical Pathology.

2015;**39**(8):1075-1084. DOI: 10.1097/pas.0000000000000453

[42] Wang W, Lie P, Guo M, He J. Risk of hepatotoxicity in cancer patients treated with immune checkpoint inhibitors: A systematic review and meta-analysis of published data. International Journal of Cancer. 2017;**141**(5):1018-1028. DOI: 10.1002/ijc.30678

[43] Huffman BM, Kottschade LA, Kamath PS, Markovic SN. Hepatotoxicity after immune checkpoint inhibitor therapy in melanoma: Natural progression and management. American Journal of Clinical Oncology. 2018;**41**(8):760-765. DOI: 10.1097/coc.0000000000000374

[44] Wolchok JD, Neyns B, Linette G, Negrier S, Lutzky J, Thomas L, et al. Ipilimumab monotherapy in patients with pretreated advanced melanoma: A randomised, double-blind, multicentre, phase 2, dose-ranging study. The Lancet Oncology. 2010;**11**(2):155-164. DOI: 10.1016/s1470-2045(09)70334-1

[45] Vento S, Cainelli F, Mirandola F, Cosco L, Di Perri G, Solbiati M, et al. Fulminant hepatitis on withdrawal of chemotherapy in carriers of hepatitis C virus. Lancet. 1996;**347**(8994):92-93. DOI: 10.1016/s0140-6736(96)90212-3

[46] Twelves C, Glynne-Jones R, Cassidy J, Schüller J, Goggin T, Roos B, et al. Effect of hepatic dysfunction due to liver metastases on the pharmacokinetics of capecitabine and its metabolites. Clinical Cancer Research. 1999;**5**(7):1696-1702

[47] Burney I. Cancer chemotherapy and biotherapy: Principles and practice. Sultan Qaboos University Medical Journal. 2011;**11**(3):424-425

[48] Lee WM. Drug-induced hepatotoxicity. The New England Journal of Medicine. 1995;**333**(17):1118-1127. DOI: 10.1056/nejm199510263331706

[49] McIntosh S, Davidson DL, O'Brien RT, Pearson HA. Methotrexate hepatotoxicity in children with leukemia. The Journal of Pediatrics. 1977;**90**(6):1019-1021. DOI: 10.1016/s0022-3476(77)80587-8

[50] Hutter RV, Shipkey FH, Tan CT, Murphy ML, Chowdhury M. Hepatic fibrosis in children with acute leukemia: A complication of therapy. Cancer. 1960;**13**:288-307. DOI: 10.1002/1097-0142(196003/04)13:2<288::aid-cncr2820130213>3.0.co;2-l

[51] Kremer JM, Lee RG, Tolman KG. Liver histology in rheumatoid arthritis patients receiving long-term methotrexate therapy. A prospective study with baseline and sequential biopsy samples. Arthritis and Rheumatism. 1989;**32**(2):121-127. DOI: 10.1002/anr.1780320202

[52] Ramadori G, Cameron S. Effects of systemic chemotherapy on the liver. Annals of Hepatology. 2010;**9**(2):133-143

[53] Erichsen C, Jönsson PE. Veno-occlusive liver disease after dacarbazine therapy (DTIC) for melanoma. Journal of Surgical Oncology. 1984;**27**(4):268-270. DOI: 10.1002/jso.2930270415

[54] Asbury RF, Rosenthal SN, Descalzi ME, Ratcliffe RL, Arseneau JC. Hepatic veno-occlusive disease due to DTIC. Cancer. 1980;**45**(10):2670-2674. DOI: 10.1002/1097-0142(19800515)45:10<2670::aid-cncr2820451031>3.0.co;2-l

[55] Stoneham S, Lennard L, Coen P, Lilleyman J, Saha V. Veno-occlusive disease in patients receiving thiopurines during maintenance therapy for childhood acute lymphoblastic leukaemia. British Journal

of Haematology. 2003;**123**(1):100-102. DOI: 10.1046/j.1365-2141.2003.04578.x

[56] DeLeve LD, Shulman HM, McDonald GB. Toxic injury to hepatic sinusoids: Sinusoidal obstruction syndrome (veno-occlusive disease). Seminars in Liver Disease. 2002;**22**(1): 27-42. DOI: 10.1055/s-2002-23204

[57] Björnsson E, Olsson R. Outcome and prognostic markers in severe drug-induced liver disease. Hepatology. 2005;**42**(2):481-489. DOI: 10.1002/hep.20800

[58] Andrade RJ, Lucena MI, Fernández MC, Pelaez G, Pachkoria K, García-Ruiz E, et al. Drug-induced liver injury: An analysis of 461 incidences submitted to the Spanish registry over a 10-year period. Gastroenterology. 2005;**129**(2):512-521. DOI: 10.1016/j.gastro.2005.05.006

[59] Ryan P, Nanji S, Pollett A, Moore M, Moulton CA, Gallinger S, et al. Chemotherapy-induced liver injury in metastatic colorectal cancer: Semiquantitative histologic analysis of 334 resected liver specimens shows that vascular injury but not steatohepatitis is associated with preoperative chemotherapy. The American Journal of Surgical Pathology. 2010;**34**(6):784-791. DOI: 10.1097/PAS.0b013e3181dc242c

[60] Rubbia-Brandt L, Audard V, Sartoretti P, Roth AD, Brezault C, Le Charpentier M, et al. Severe hepatic sinusoidal obstruction associated with oxaliplatin-based chemotherapy in patients with metastatic colorectal cancer. Annals of Oncology. 2004;**15**(3):460-466. DOI: 10.1093/annonc/mdh095

[61] Valla DC, Cazals-Hatem D. Sinusoidal obstruction syndrome. Clinics and Research in Hepatology and Gastroenterology. 2016;**40**(4):378-385. DOI: 10.1016/j.clinre.2016.01.006

[62] Fan CQ, Crawford JM. Sinusoidal obstruction syndrome (hepatic veno-occlusive disease). Journal of Clinical and Experimental Hepatology. 2014;**4**(4):332-346. DOI: 10.1016/j.jceh.2014.10.002

[63] Hudis CA. Trastuzumab—mechanism of action and use in clinical practice. The New England Journal of Medicine. 2007;**357**(1):39-51. DOI: 10.1056/NEJMra043186

[64] Pritchard J, McElwain TJ, Graham-Pole J. High-dose melphalan with autologous marrow for treatment of advanced neuroblastoma. British Journal of Cancer. 1982;**45**(1):86-94. DOI: 10.1038/bjc.1982.11

[65] Hoy SM, Lyseng-Williamson KA. Intravenous Busulfan. Pediatric Drugs. 2007;**9**(4):271-278. DOI: 10.2165/00148581-200709040-00008

[66] Zhou H, Wang YX, Lou HY, Xu XJ, Zhang MM. Hepatic sinusoidal obstruction syndrome caused by herbal medicine: CT and MRI features. Korean Journal of Radiology. 2014;**15**(2):218-225. DOI: 10.3348/kjr.2014.15.2.218

[67] Shin NY, Kim MJ, Lim JS, Park MS, Chung YE, Choi JY, et al. Accuracy of gadoxetic acid-enhanced magnetic resonance imaging for the diagnosis of sinusoidal obstruction syndrome in patients with chemotherapy-treated colorectal liver metastases. European Radiology. 2012;**22**(4):864-871. DOI: 10.1007/s00330-011-2333-x

[68] Weber JS, Yang JC, Atkins MB, Disis ML. Toxicities of immunotherapy for the practitioner. Journal of Clinical Oncology. 2015;**33**(18):2092-2099. DOI: 10.1200/jco.2014.60.0379

[69] Gangi A, Lu SC. Chemotherapy-associated liver injury in colorectal cancer. Therapeutic Advances in Gastroenterology. 2020;**13**:1756284820924194. DOI: 10.1177/1756284820924194

[70] Langley RE, Gilbert DC, Duong T, Clarke NW, Nankivell M, Rosen SD, et al. Transdermal oestradiol for androgen suppression in prostate cancer: Long-term cardiovascular outcomes from the randomised prostate adenocarcinoma transcutaneous hormone (PATCH) trial programme. Lancet. 2021;**397**(10274):581-591. DOI: 10.1016/s0140-6736(21)00100-8

Chapter 3

Paracetamol-Induced Hepatotoxicity

Nida Mirza

Abstract

Drug-induced hepatotoxicity is common in clinical settings, one of the commonly used drugs leading to liver injury is paracetamol. It is a commonly used analgesic and antipyretic drug. The toxicity of paracetamol has been described in accidental, iatrogenic, and intentional ingestion; also, the extent of liver injury varies from person to person depending on host factors, nutritional status, age, etc. The toxicity of paracetamol is not usually recognized by clinicians as initially, the symptoms are subtle. There is a specific antidote available for paracetamol-induced liver injury to prevent acute liver failure; however, it needs to be given time for proper action, therefore a strong clinical suspicion is to be taken when there is no proper history of ingestion.

Keywords: paracetamol, N-acetyl cysteine, drug-induced liver injury

1. Introduction

The liver contributes significantly to the metabolism and removal of drugs from the human body [1]. Metabolization of drugs and xenobiotics to nontoxic substances in the liver by enzymes is important for the proper function of the body, alteration in these statuses leads to a shift of metabolism toward the production of oxidants, which coheres to lipids or nuclear proteins which results in mutations, membrane damage, and alteration of enzyme activity respectively which further leads to organ malfunction. The production of oxidants is the most common action in the pathogenesis of liver damage by pharmaceutical drugs and herbal products [2]. Liver damage may occur due to environmental toxicants, drugs, and microbial metabolites. There are two sets of enzymes, phase I and phase II enzymes which play a very important role in the metabolism and detoxification of various drugs and other toxins. Paracetamol is one of the most commonly used drugs as an analgesic and antipyretic, it is a structural analog of phenacetin, which was withdrawn due to concerns for nephrotoxicity. Paracetamol is relatively safe compared with other NSAIDS; however, overdose can cause a spectrum of liver injuries from mild elevation in liver enzymes to acute liver failure and encephalopathy [3]. A lot of research has been conducted to know the pathogenesis of paracetamol-induced liver toxicity. N-acetyl cysteine (NAC) is used as an antidote for paracetamol-overdosed patients; however, it should be administered as early as possible [4]. It has now been recognized that paracetamol toxicity consists of multiple pathways, including paracetamol metabolism, oxidative stress, endoplasmic reticulum stress, autophagy, sterile inflammation, microcirculatory dysfunction, and compensatory liver repair and regeneration. Some patients with liver failure require liver transplantation for survival [5]. In this chapter, we have discussed the paracetamol-induced hepatotoxicity, pathophysiology, and factors that increase the risk of its toxicity, prevention, treatment, and patient outcome.

2. Epidemiology and pathogenesis

2.1 Incidence of hepatotoxicity

Paracetamol overdose is among one of the commonest causes of acute liver failure in some countries. The common settings for paracetamol-induced liver injury are suicidal overdose, unintentionally or accidentally in alcoholics, and with therapeutic use [6]. Studies done in the adult population have shown the most common etiology of acute liver failure (40%) was paracetamol overdose, more with unintentional intake rather than taken for suicide [7, 8]. However, a multicenter prospective study of pediatric patients reported that only 14% of acute liver failure is attributed to paracetamol overdose [9]. In a study on patients with an unintentional overdose of narcotic users, around 30% of patients were also taking over-the-counter paracetamol along with narcotic drugs. Patients sometimes are not knowing that their pain-reliving medicines advised by a physician are in combination with paracetamol and thus may take these medications along with oral over-the-counter paracetamol resulting in overdose. Due to delayed presentation and treatment, risk of mortality is comparatively more with unintentional overdose rather than intentional overdosage [10]. In 19% and 12.5% of indeterminate ALF, paracetamol-protein adducts were identified [11, 12]. In chronic alcoholics, paracetamol-induced hepatotoxicity has been well recognized and reported to occur at lower doses compared with non-alcoholics [13, 14]. In a study on chronic alcoholics with paracetamol hepatotoxicity, the average toxic dose of paracetamol was 7 g per day; however, a lower dose of 2.5 g per day has also found to cause toxicity [15]. Paracetamol hepatotoxicity had been found with ingestion of therapeutic doses in individuals with malnutrition, advanced age, chronic pulmonary diseases, cardiac dysfunction, and chronic liver disease [16]. Drug interactions of paracetamol with other drugs (e.g., anticonvulsants, antitubercular) also result in hepatotoxicity at lower doses [17, 18].

2.2 Toxic dose in adults and children

In single oral ingestion, the toxic dose for children is more than 200 mg/kg of body weight, whereas in adults and adolescents, it is more than 7.5 g. In children younger than 6 years of age, toxicity occurs after ingestion of more than 75 mg/kg body weight per day. Acute toxic dose is in a single dose in repeated dosing [19], However, toxic dose also varies in different ethical groups like in Japanese lower doses may cause intoxication [20]. Children are found to be less sensitive to acute intoxication than adults, and this may be due to larger glutathione stores and comparatively larger liver [21].

2.3 Pathophysiology

Paracetamol enters the enterohepatic circulation after absorption in the gut and the liver by glucuronidation and sulfation 95% of its metabolized, and only a small amount of the drug is removed by the kidneys. In therapeutic doses, 2.7 hours is the mean elimination half-life of paracetamol ingestion [22]. N-acetyl-p-benzoquinone

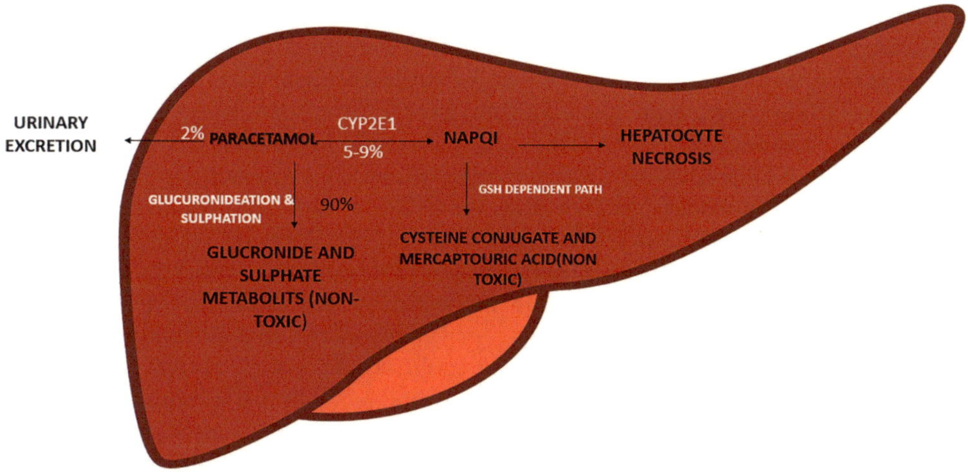

Figure 1.
Metabolism of paracetamol.

imine (NAPQI) is formed by oxidation reaction in approximately 5% fraction of the drug, and this further binds to cysteine, DNA, and lipids. Antioxidant glutathione (GSH) detoxifies NAPQI by forming a mercapturic metabolite, which is removed by the kidneys (**Figure 1**). On ingestion of a higher dose of paracetamol, intracellular GSH is depleted and there is a relative shunting of the metabolism of paracetamol toward oxidation, thus forming increased amounts of NAPQI. CYP2E1 has a primary role in the oxidation of paracetamol; however, some other CYP isoforms have been identified, including CYP3A4 and CYP1A2. A major portion of CYP2E1 is distributed in the centrilobular regions of the hepatic lobule, leading to centrilobular necrosis as seen on biopsy [23]. The greatest intrinsic activity toward paracetamol is of CYP2E1 and CYP3A among all known CYPs. Studies conducted in the mouse model of paracetamol overdose showed paracetamol adduct formation occurs in centrilobular hepatocytes [24] liver biopsy if done, the histopathology of liver tissue shows centrizonal necrosis and mild inflammation [25]. The main autopsy finding in those who died due to liver failure is centrizonal hemorrhagic necrosis with no or little inflammatory reaction and normal histologic appearance of portal tracts [26].

3. Clinical manifestations and laboratory findings

Paracetamol overdose identification is of significant value as an early start of treatment can prevent morbidity and mortality significantly. Many a times, patients may not tell the information about paracetamol ingestion and exact dosage. The most common symptoms are malaise, nausea with/without vomiting, and abdominal pain, as these symptoms are not peculiar leading to difficulty in making the diagnosis in absence of a history of overdose. The clinical course of paracetamol hepatotoxicity has four established sequential phases [27]. Each phase usually occurs following a fixed time interval after the paracetamol over-ingestion; however, these may be modified by factors like the formulation (mixed with opiate preparations, sustained release, etc.), co-ingestion (alcohol, herbal supplements, or other pharmaceutical drugs), and presence of chronic liver disease. The first phase starts within the first

24 hours of intake of the drug and usually has symptoms such as nausea, vomiting, muscle aches, dullness, and perspiration. However, some patients may remain asymptomatic in this phase, which leads to a delay in the diagnosis in patients who are unaware of their overdose. Biochemically liver transaminase values are usually normal in this phase. In the second phase that occurs 24 hours to 72 hours after intake, transaminases and bilirubin begin to rise and prothrombin time may be prolonged [28, 29]. Liver transaminase [alanine aminotransferase (ALT) and aspartate aminotransferase (AST)] may rise to several thousand IU [30]. There are lesser increases in alkaline phosphatase and bilirubin. In phase III that occurs 72 hours to 96 hours after ingestion, liver injury occurs maximally in this phase and is characterized by continued progression of hepatotoxicity, possibly fulminant hepatic failure, and the onset of multiorgan system failure and hypoglycemia, jaundice, oliguria, acute tubular necrosis, encephalopathy, coagulopathy and lactic acidosis, central nervous system symptoms including confusion, somnolence, or coma. The risk of mortality is maximum in the third phase, mostly due to multi-organ dysfunction. There is a "two-hit" mechanism in the development of lactic acidosis one is that NAPQI in excess causes mitochondrial dysregulation, which is further followed subsequently by tissue hypoxia and decreased hepatic metabolism and clearance of lactate [8, 31]. Phase IV occurs after approximately 96 hours after the recovery from the third phase, the patient may either die from liver failure and its complications or start to recover. Those who improve liver functions usually return to normal within three weeks, with the histological improvement of the liver within 3 months. Usually, the fourth phase lasts for 1 to 2 weeks, but its duration varies from patient to patient. Aminotransferase elevations usually resolve within two weeks duration. An early signal of severe toxicity is prolonged prothrombin time within 30-hour of paracetamol ingestion [32]. Usually, bilirubin levels do not go higher as compared with liver failure due to other etiology [33]. Acute renal failure may occur in association with hepatotoxicity and also can occur as the liver injury is improving and some may even need dialysis [34–36]. A distinguished feature of paracetamol overdose in chronic alcoholics is seen in which laboratory abnormalities may include extremely high serum aminotransferase levels (AST > ALT) and prolonged prothrombin time within a small time frame of ingestion [37].

3.1 Kings college criteria

King's College criteria are used for mortality prediction in ALF caused by paracetamol. The criteria include the presence of metabolic acidosis (arterial pH < 7.30) alone OR the presence of these three: Grade III or IV hepatic encephalopathy (HE), prothrombin time (PT) > 100 sec, and creatinine level > 3.4 mg/dL [38].

4. Treatment

4.1 General management

On assessment of paracetamol overdose, a detailed history should be taken, which should include ingested dose, co-intake of other pharmaceutical drugs or herbal medications, alcohol intake (acute and chronic), presence of any liver disease or disorder, and any other co-morbidity. Biochemical parameters including serum AST,

ALT, bilirubin, prothrombin time, blood urea nitrogen (BUN), creatinine, electrolytes, complete blood count, and urinalysis should be done. The plasma paracetamol levels should be sent for measurement ideally 4 hours after ingestion or as early as 24 hours, but not before 4 hours because continuous absorption of paracetamol leads to falsely low levels. The test should be repeated after 4 hours of the first test and then at 16, 24, and 32 hours after ingestion. Management for paracetamol overdose includes prevention of absorption from the gut, elimination of absorbed paracetamol from the blood, inhibition of formation of toxic metabolite NAPQI, and detoxification of NAPQI. The timing of presentation and the degree of hepatic decompensation guide the choice of therapy. Gastric lavage, administration of activated charcoal, and ipecacuanha (induces emesis) can prevent or decrease gut absorption within the first few hours after ingestion [39, 40]. NAC is used as an antidote in paracetamol overdose, and if initiated within the first 8 hours from the time of ingestion or overdose, a good response is seen. Methionine and cysteamine also cause detoxification of NAPQI, but have shown severe adverse central nervous system effects so not used commonly [41]. It has been found that starting NAC therapy as late as 36 hours after overdose leads to a significantly better outcome in paracetamol hepatotoxicity [42]. NAC acts by restoring glutathione levels (hydrolyzed to cysteine, which restores glutathione), attaching to NAPQI and by increasing conjugation reaction in hepatocytes leading to the formation of non-toxic products [43]. Mortality from paracetamol overdose had declined from 5% without the use of antidote to 0.7% with the use of NAC. Cimetidine was used initially to prevent the formation of NAPQI as it inhibits cytochrome P450 but was not effective in many trials [44, 45]. Liver transplantation should be considered to prevent mortality in selected cases.

4.2 N-acetylcysteine

The standard dosage of oral NAC is a single dose of 140 mg per kg and after that 17 doses of 70 mg per kg over 72 hours. The total dose thus will be 1330 mg/kg. The standard dosage of intravenous NAC is typically three weight-based doses; the first dose is 150 mg per kg in the first 1 hour, the second dose is 50 mg per kg to be given over 4 hours, and lastly, third dose is 100 mg per kg to be given over 16 hours [46]. Higher hepatic concentrations can be achieved by oral NAC therapy, and the only issue is that it is unpalatable, also difficult for children to consume so many doses, and may cause vomiting. Intravenous N-acetylcysteine therapy results in higher plasma concentrations and is more convenient for those who are vomiting; side effects of parentally given NAC can be an allergic reaction, which is mostly mild and treated by antihistaminics and by temporarily stopping intravenous NAC [47].

4.3 The Rumack: Matthew nomogram

The Rumack–Matthew nomogram is the semilogarithmic plot of plasma paracetamol levels with time and is used to assess potential hepatotoxicity. This nomogram was developed retrospectively based on data from patients who has single paracetamol overdose and acute ingestions of paracetamol and had not received treatment with the antidote. The nomogram forecasts potential toxicity from 4 hours to 24 hours following ingestion. The upper line of the nomogram is the "probable" line, also known as the Rumack–Matthew line (**Figure 2**). Around two-third of a patient with paracetamol levels above this line will have a liver injury. The lower line is the

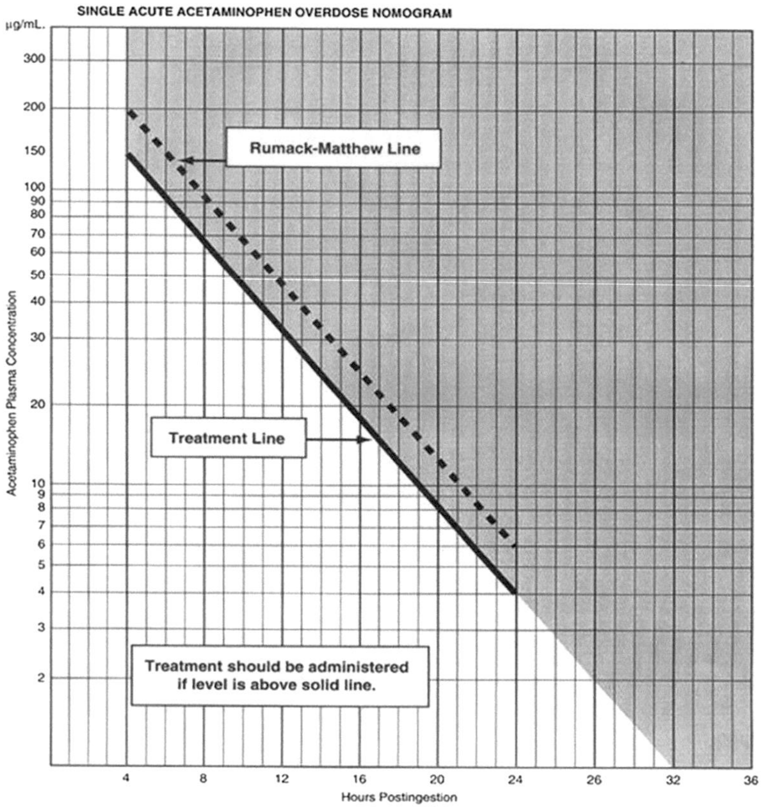

Figure 2.
Rumack–Matthew nomogram: Serum paracetamol concentration vs. time post ingestion. Taken from Rumack and Matthew [48].

"possible" line and includes a 25% margin of error in level estimation discrepancy or unreliable ingestion time. Using the Rumack–Matthew nomogram patients treated with supportive care only who had paracetamol levels above the probable hepatic toxicity line had a 14–89% incidence of hepatotoxicity and a mortality of 5–24% [49, 50]. Poor prognostic signs identified are age group >50 years a plasma factor V concentration < 10% of normal [51].

4.4 N-acetylcysteine dosing and Rumack–Matthew nomogram

In a case of single ingestion of paracetamol overdose, obtain paracetamol concentration at as early as possible but not before 4 hours. If the paracetamol concentration on the Rumack–Matthew nomogram is above the "treatment line" (the line connecting 150 μg/mL [993 μmol/L] at 4 hours and 4.7 μg/mL [31 μmol/L] at 24 hours), administration of NAC is indicated. If time of ingestion is not known exactly, then it is less than 24 hours post-ingestion NAC should be started, if plotted above treatment line. In a case where patient has ingested extended-release formulations or co-ingested with other drugs like opioids, anticholinergics, or other medications that slows gut motility, if the initial 4-hour concentration plots above the treatment line, NAC should be initiated within 8 hours post-ingestion [52].

4.5 Management for acute liver failure

Acute liver failure is defined as severe acute liver injury for fewer than 26-week duration with encephalopathy and impaired synthetic function (INR >1.5 or higher) in a patient without pre-existing liver disease. ALF can lead to multiorgan dysfunction, which can present as hypotension, acute renal failure, coagulopathy, encephalopathy, sepsis, and cerebral edema. Intensive care is needed for patient with acute liver failure as they may deteriorate rapidly. A proper centra venous line and arterial line for hemodynamic monitoring and, as well as a urinary catheter for urine output monitoring. Coagulation parameters, blood counts, metabolic panels, blood sugar, and arterial blood gases are to be measured with proper time intervals. The neurological status should be evaluated regularly, for cerebral edema and intracranial pressure monitoring when intracranial hypertension is identified [53, 54]. Patient should be admitted in intensive care unit in presence of encephalopathy and coagulopathy. Due to risk of rapid deterioration, a proper communication with liver transplant centers should be done and transfer decisions should be considered for those who had rising INR, rising creatinine or decreasing urine output, metabolic acidosis, hypotension, or/and encephalopathy [55]. Retrospective study showed treatment after 10–36 hours with NAC was associated with a mortality of 37% when compared with 58% in patients given supportive treatment only, while prospective study with 50 patients with established liver failure showed mortality was 20% in the treated group versus 48% ($P < 0.05$) in the controls [56, 57]. Liver transplantation is another therapeutic option for patients with paracetamol-induced fulminant hepatic failure. Early recognition of poor prognostic factors can be useful in determining need for transplant and providing time to obtain a donor. Many factors affect survival, and the development of ALF after paracetamol overdose ALF in pediatric patients had 100% survival with grade II, but only 18% with grade III, also the development of cerebral edema reduced survival to 22% [58]. Significantly better survival is reported for patients who sought medical care within 24 hours of ingestion compared with later presentation. The overall mortality is as high as 28% for patients who develop ALF from paracetamol overdose, which is better than rates for ALF due to other causes. Reported survival rates for paracetamol-induced ALF vary from 65–73% without liver transplantation. Requirement of inotropic support is a poor survival factor and survival rate is below 10% in patients with metabolic acidosis that failed to respond to adequate fluid resuscitation [59]. Serum creatinine concentrations and PT are closely correlated with survival. Survival rate of 80% patients for peak PT below 90 seconds, which reduces to 8% around for PT beyond 180 seconds [60]. Survival rate is around 65% for patients with serum creatinine below 100 mmol/L, which reduces to 23% if above 300 mmol/L. Requirement of liver transplantation was less in paracetamol-induced ALF than ALF due to other causes [61]. In a recent study, overall survival rate after liver transplantation was about 70%, with 1-year survival of 73% after 1 year and 67% at the end of 5 years. Multiorgan failure and neurologic complications are attributed for most of the deaths after liver transplantation [62].

5. Conclusion

The morbidity and mortality from paracetamol overdose vary from patient to patient, and also depend on underlying comorbidities, nutritional status, history of alcoholism and co ingestion of other drugs. Overdose nay result in mild liver injury, clinically significant hepatotoxicity, or death, and timely administration of antidote directs prognosis. Death from paracetamol overdose in developed countries has decreased to 1–2% after the use of N-Acetyl cysteine, which was previously much higher (6–25%).

Conflict of interest

The authors declare no conflict of interest.

Author details

Nida Mirza
Sri Aurbindo Institute of Medical Science, Indore, India

*Address all correspondence to: nydamirza.1@gmail.com

References

[1] Pandit A, Sachdeva T, Bafna P. Drug-induced hepatotoxicity: A review. Journal of Applied Pharmaceutical Science. 2012;**02**:233-243. DOI: 10.7324/japs.2012.2541

[2] Upadhyay G, Gupta SP, Prakash O, Singh MP. Pyrogallol-mediated toxicity and natural antioxidants: Triumphs and pitfalls of preclinical findings and their translational limitations. Chemico-Biological Interactions. 2010a;**183**:333-340. DOI: 10.1016/j.cbi.2009.11.028

[3] Jacqz-Aigrain E, Anderson BJ. Pain control: Non-steroidal anti-inflammatory agents. Seminars in Fetal & Neonatal Medicine. 2006;**11**:251-259. DOI: 10.1016/j.siny.2006.02.009

[4] Jeong HH, Cha K, Choi KH, et al. Evaluation of cut-off values in acute paracetamol overdose following the United Kingdom guidelines. BMC Pharmacology and Toxicology. 2022;**23**:5. DOI: 10.1186/s40360-021-00547-1

[5] Food and Drug Administration, HHS. Organ-specific warnings; internal analgesic, antipyretic, and antirheumatic drug products for over-the-counter human use; final monograph. Final rule. Federal Register. 2009 Apr 29;**74**(81):19385-19409. PMID: 19507324

[6] Smilkstein MJ, Knapp GL, Kulig KW, Rumack BH. Efficacy of oral *N*acetyl cysteine in the treatment of acetaminophen overdose. Analysis of the national multicenter study (1976 to 1988). The New England Journal of Medicine. 1988;**319**:1557-1562

[7] Bernal W. Changing patterns of causation and the use of transplantation in the United Kingdom. Seminars in Liver Disease. 2003;**23**:227-237

[8] Ostapowicz G, Fontana RJ, Schiødt FV, et al. Results of a prospective study of acute liver failure at 17 tertiary care centers in the United States. Annals of Internal Medicine. 2002;**137**:947-954

[9] Bower WA, Johns M, Margolis HS, et al. Population-based surveillance for acute liver failure. The American Journal of Gastroenterology. 2007;**102**:2459-2463

[10] Squires RH, Shneider BL, Bucuvalas J, et al. Acute liver failure in children: The first 348 patients in the pediatric acute liver failure study group. The Journal of Pediatrics. 2006;**148**:652-658

[11] Schiødt FV, Rochling FA, Casey DL, et al. Acetaminophen toxicity in an urban county hospital. The New England Journal of Medicine. 1997;**337**:1112-1117

[12] Davern TJ II, James LP, Hinson JA, et al. Measurement of serum acetaminophen-protein adducts in patients with acute liver failure. Gastroenterology. 2006;**130**:687-694

[13] McClain CJ, Holtzman J, Allen J, Kromhout J, Shedlofsky S. Clinical features of acetaminophen toxicity. Journal of Clinical Gastroenterology. 1988;**10**:76-80

[14] Maddrey WC. Hepatic effects of acetaminophen. Enhanced toxicity in alcoholics. Journal of Clinical Gastroenterology. 1987;**9**:180-185

[15] Seifert CF, Lucas DS, Vondracek TG, Kastens DJ, McCarty DL, Bui B. Patterns of acetaminophen use in alcoholic patients. Pharmacotherapy. 1993;**13**:391-395

[16] Bonkovsky HL, Kane RE, Jones DP, Galinsky RE, Banner B. Acute hepatic

and renal toxicity from low doses of acetaminophen in the absence of alcohol abuse or malnutrition: Evidence for increased susceptibility to drug toxicity due to cardiopulmonary and renal insufficiency. Hepatology. 1994;**19**:1141-1148

[17] Bonkovsky HL, Mudge GH, McMurty RJ. Chronic hepatic inflammation and fibrosis due to low doses of parcetamol. Lancet. 1978;**1**:1016-1018

[18] Crippin JS. Acetaminophen hepatotoxicity: Potentiation by isoniazid. The American Journal of Gastroenterology. 1993;**88**:590-592

[19] Heard K et al. Toxicity from repeated doses of acetaminophen in children: Assessment of causality and dose in reported cases. American Journal of Therapeutics. 2014;**21**(3):174-183

[20] Washio M, Inoue N. The risk factors of death from the acetaminophen poisoning with antipyretic-analgesic drugs in Japan. Fukuoka Igaku Zasshi. 1997;**88**(11):352-357

[21] Bond GR. Reduced toxicity of acetaminophen in children: It's the liver. Journal of Toxicology. Clinical Toxicology. 2004;**42**(2):149-152

[22] Janes J, Routledge PA. Recent developments in the management of paracetamol (acetaminophen) poisoning. Drug Safety. 1992;7:170-177

[23] Thummel KE, Lee CA, Kunze KL, Nelson SD, Slattery JT. Oxidation of acetaminophen to N-acetyl-p-aminobenzoquinoneimine by human CYP3A4. Biochemical Pharmacology. 1993;**45**:1563-1569

[24] Patten CJ, Thomas PE, Guy RL, Lee M, Gonzalez FJ, Guengerich FP, et al. Cytochrome P450 enzymes involved in acetaminophen activation by rat and human liver microsomes and their kinetics. Chemical Research in Toxicology. 1993;**6**:511-518

[25] Prescott LF, Illingworth RN, Critchley JA, Stewart MJ, Adam RD, Proudfoot AT. Intravenous N-acetylcystine: The treatment of choice for paracetamol poisoning. British Medical Journal. 1979;**2**:1097-1100. DOI: 10.1136/bmj.2.6198.1097

[26] Seeff LB, Cuccherini BA, Zimmerman HJ, Adler E, Benjamin SB. Acetaminophenhepatotoxicityinalcoholics. A therapeutic misadventure. Annals of Internal Medicine. 1986;**104**:399-404

[27] Pumford NR, Hinson JA, Potter DW, Rowland KL, Benson RW, Roberts DW. Immunochemical quantitation of 3-(cystein-S-yl) acetaminophen adducts in serum and liver proteins of acetaminophen-treated mice. The Journal of Pharmacology and Experimental Therapeutics. 1989;**248**:190-196

[28] Watkins PB, Kaplowitz N, Slattery JT, Colonese CR, Colucci SV, Stewart PW, et al. Aminotransferase elevations in healthy adults receiving 4 grams of acetaminophen daily: A randomized controlled trial. JAMA. 2006;**296**:87-93

[29] Jaeschke H, McGill MR. Cytochrome P450-derived versus mitochondrial oxidant stress in acetaminophen hepatotoxicity. Toxicology Letters. 2015;**235**:216-217. DOI: 10.1016/j.toxlet.2015.04.002

[30] Rumack BH. Acetaminophen overdose in children and adolescents. Pediatric Clinics of North America. 1986;**33**:691-701

[31] McGill MR, Sharpe MR, Williams CD, Taha M, Curry SC,

Jaeschke H. The mechanism underlying acetaminophen-induced hepatotoxicity in humans and mice involves mitochondrial damage and nuclear DNA fragmentation. The Journal of Clinical Investigation. 2012;**122**:1574-1583. DOI: 10.1172/JCI59755

[32] Singer AJ, Carracio TR, Mofenson HC. The temporal profile of increased transaminase levels in patients with acetaminophen-induced liver dysfunction. Annals of Emergency Medicine. 1995;**26**:4953

[33] Gazzard BG, Henderson JM, Williams R. Early changes in coagulation following a paracetamol overdose and a controlled trial of fresh frozen plasma therapy. Gut. 1975;**16**:617-620

[34] Thornton JR, Losowsky MS. Severe thrombocytopenia after paracetamol overdose. Gut. 1990;**31**:1159-1160

[35] Boyer TD, Rouff SL. Acetaminophen-induced hepatic necrosis and renal failure. JAMA. 1971;**218**:440-441

[36] Khandelwal N, James L, Sanders C, Larson AM, Lee WM, The Acute Liver Failure Study Group. Unrecognized acetaminophen toxicity as a cause of "indeterminate" acute liver failure. Hepatology. 2011;**53**:567-576

[37] Prescott LF. Effects of non-narcotic analgesics on the liver. Drugs. 1986;**32**(Suppl. 4):129-147

[38] O'Grady JG, Alexander GJM, Hayllar KM, Williams R. Early indicators of prognosis in fulminant hepatic failure. Gastroenterology. 1989;**97**:439-445

[39] Brok J, Buckley N, Gluud C. Interventions for paracetamol (acetaminophen) overdose. Cochrane Database of Systematic Reviews. 2006:CD003328

[40] Underhill TJ, Greene MK, Dove AF. A comparison of the efficacy of gastric lavage, ipecacuanha and activated charcoal in the emergency management of paracetamol overdose. Archives of Emergency Medicine. 1990;7:148-154

[41] Greene SL, Dargan PI, Jones AL. Acute poisoning: Understanding 90% of cases in a nutshell. Postgraduate Medical Journal. 2005;**81**:204-216

[42] Bateman DN, Dear JW. Acetylcysteine in paracetamol poisoning: A perspective of 45 years of use. Toxicology Research. 2019;**8**(4):489-498. DOI: 10.1039/c9tx00002j

[43] Heard KJ. Acetylcysteine for acetaminophen poisoning. The New England Journal of Medicine. 2008;**359**:285-292. DOI: 10.1056/NEJMct0708278

[44] Kerr F, Dawson A, Whyte IM, Buckley N, Murray L, Graudins A, et al. The Australasian Clinical Toxicology Investigators Collaboration randomized trial of different loading infusion rates of N- acetylcysteine. Annals of Emergency Medicine. 2005;**45**:402-408. DOI: 10.1016/j.annemergmed.2004.08.040

[45] Burkhart KK, Janco N, Kulig KW, et al. Cimetidine as adjunctive treatment for acetaminophen overdose. Human & Experimental Toxicology. 1995;**14**:299-304

[46] Rumack BH. Acetaminophen hepatotoxicity: The first 35 years. Journal of Toxicology. Clinical Toxicology. 2002;**40**:3-20. DOI: 10.1081/CLT-120002882

[47] Schenker S, Maddrey WC. Subliminal drug-drug interactions: Users and their physicians take notice. Hepatology. 1991;**13**:995-998

[48] Rumack BH, Matthew H. Acetaminophen poisoning and toxicity. Pediatrics. 1975;**55**(6):871-876

[49] Prescott LF. Paracetamol overdosage. Pharmacological considerations and clinical management. Drugs. 1983;**25**:290-314

[50] Rotundo L, Pyrsopoulos N. Liver injury induced by paracetamol and challenges associated with intentional and unintentional use. World Journal of Hepatology. 2020;**12**(4):125-136. DOI: 10.4254/wjh.v12.i4.125

[51] Ml S, Bronstein AC, Linden C, Augenstein WL, Kulig KW, Rumack BH. Acetaminophen overdose: A 48-hour intravenous N-acetylcysteine treatment protocol. Annals of Emergency Medicine. 1991;**20**(1058-61):063

[52] Jones AL. Mechanism of action and value of N-acetylcysteine in the treatment of early and late acetaminophen poisoning: A critical review. Journal of Toxicology. Clinical Toxicology. 1998;**36**:277-285

[53] Salgia AD, Kosnik SD. When acetaminophen use becomes toxic. Treating acute accidental and intentional overdose. Postgraduate Medicine. 1999;**105**:81-90

[54] Rinella ME, Sanyal A. Intensive management of hepatic failure. Seminars in Respiratory and Critical Care Medicine. 2006;**27**:241-261

[55] Stravitz RT, Kramer AH, Davern T, et al. Intensive care of patients with acute liver failure: Recommendations of the U.S. Acute Liver Failure Study Group. Critical Care Medicine. 2007;**35**:2498-2508

[56] Harrison PM, Keays R, Bray GP, Alexander GJM, Williams R. Improved outcome of paracetamol-induced fulminant hepatic failure by late administration of acetylcysteine. Lancet. 1990a;**335**:1572-1573

[57] Keays R, Harrison PM, Wendon JA, Forbes A, Gove C. Alexander GJM, Williams R. Intravenous acetylcysteine in paracetamol induced fulminant hepatic failure: A prospective controlled trial. BMJ. 1991;**303**:1026-1029

[58] Makin AJ, Wendon J, Williams R. A 7-year experience of severe acetaminophen-induced hepatotoxicity (1987-1993). Gastroenterology. 1995;**109**:1907-1916

[59] Makin AJ, Williams R. Acetaminophen-induced hepatotoxicity: Predisposing factors and treatments. Advances in Internal Medicine. 1997;**42**:453-483

[60] Harrison PM, O'Grady JG, Keays RT, et al. Serial prothrom- bin time as prognostic indicator in paracetamol induced fulminant hepatic failure. BMJ. 1990;**301**:964-966

[61] Bernal W, Wendon J, Rela M, et al. Use and outcome of liver transplantation in acetaminophen-induced acute liver failure. Hepatology. 1998;**27**:1050-1055

[62] Farmer DG, Anselmo DM, Ghobrial RM, et al. Liver transplantation for fulminant hepatic failure: Experience with more than 200 patients over a 17-year period. Annals of Surgery. 2003;**237**:666-675

Chapter 4

Radiation Induced Liver Toxicity

Debnarayan Dutta and Yarlagadda Sreenija

Abstract

Liver was always considered to be 'highly sensitive' to radiation therapy (RT) and was not considered 'safe' for radiation therapy treatment. The most significant radiation induced liver toxicity was described by Ingold et al. as "Radiation hepatitis." Historically, radiation to liver lesions with curative intent or incidental exposure during adjacent organ treatment or total body irradiation implied whole organ irradiation due to lack of high precision technology. Whole organ irradiation led to classic clinical picture termed as "Radiation Induced Liver Disease (RILD)." In conventional fractionation, the whole liver could be treated only to the doses of 30–35Gy safely, which mostly serves as palliation rather than cure. With the advent of technological advancements like IMRT, especially stereotactic radiation therapy (SBRT), the notion of highly precise and accurate treatment has been made practically possible. The toxicity profile for this kind of focused radiation was certainly different from that of whole organ irradiation. There have been attempts made to characterize the effects caused by the high precision radiation. Thus, the QUANTEC liver paper distinguished RILD to 'classic' and 'non-classic' types. *Classic RILD* is defined as 'anicteric hepatomegaly and ascites', and also can also have elevated alkaline phosphatase (more than twice the upper limit of normal or baseline value). This is the type of clinical picture encountered following irradiation of whole or greater part of the organ. *Non-classic RILD* is defined by elevated liver transaminases more than five times the upper limit of normal or a decline in liver function (measured by a worsening of Child-Pugh score by 2 or more), in the absence of classic RILD. In patients with baseline values more than five times the upper limit of normal, CTCAE Grade 4 levels are within 3 months after completion of RT. This is the type of RILD that is encountered typically after high-dose radiation to a smaller part of liver. It is commonly associated with infective etiology. Emami et al. reported the liver tolerance doses or TD 5/5 (5% complication rate in 5 years) as 50 Gy for one-third (33%) of the liver, 35 Gy for two-thirds (67%) of the liver, and 30 Gy for the whole liver (100%). Liver function (Child Pugh Score), infective etiology, performance status and co-morbidities influence the radiation induced toxicity. Lyman–Kutcher–Burman (LKB)-NTCP model was used to assess dose-volume risk of RILD. Lausch et al. at London Regional Cancer Program (LRCP), developed a logistic TCP model. Quantitative Analysis of Normal Tissue Effects in the Clinic (QUANTEC) reported recommendations that mean normal liver dose should be <18 Gy for baseline CP-A patients and < 6 Gy for those with CP-B, for a 6-fraction SBRT regimen. The University of Colorado phase 1 clinical trial of SBRT for liver metastases described the importance of the liver volume spared, that is, 'critical volume model.' It is estimated that a typical normal liver volume is approximately 2000 mL and specified that a minimum volume of 700 mL or 35% of normal liver should remain uninjured by SBRT i.e. at least 700 mL of normal liver (entire liver minus cumulative GTV) had to receive at total dose less than 15 Gy. In treatment regimen of 48 Gy in 3 fractions, CP-A patients were required to either limit the dose to 33% of the uninvolved liver (D33%) < 10 Gy and maintain the liver volume receiving <7 Gy to <500 cc. In more conservative treatment regimen, such as in 40 Gy in 5 fractions schedule, CP-B7 patients had to meet constraints of D33% < 18 Gy and/or > 500 cc receiving <12 Gy. The concept of body surface area (BSA) and Basal Metabolic Index (BMI) guided estimation of optimal liver volume is required to estimate the liver volume need to be spared during SBRT treatment. Radiation induced liver injury is potentially hazardous complication. There is no definitive treatment and a proportion of patient may land up in gross decompensation. Usually supportive care, diuretics, albumin supplement, and vitamin K replacement may be useful. Better case selection will avert incidence of RILD. Precise imaging, contouring, planning and respecting normal tissue constraints are critical. Radiation delivery with motion management and image guidance will allow delivery of higher dose and spare normal liver and hence will improve response to treatment and reduce RILD.

Keywords: liver, toxicity, radiation therapy, RILD, SBRT, cyberknife, radiation therapy

1. Introduction

Liver was always considered to be 'highly sensitive' to radiation therapy and was not considered 'safe' for radiation therapy treatment. For many years, maximal tolerable dose (mean liver dose) for liver was considered to be low and radiation dose required for therapeutic effect for liver tumors (Hepatocellular carcinoma, Cholangiocarcinoma) was considered high. Hence, radiation therapy was mostly not considered for liver tumors. Liver is a moving organ and movement of liver is dependent on many factors such as breathing pattern, stomach filling, peristaltic movements, and hence liver movement is not predictable. There were no appropriate tracking technology or high dose radiation delivery technology in 'moving' targets like liver. Hence, in early years of radiation therapy there are only a few anecdotal reports of radiation therapy delivery in liver tumors. In recent years, with advent of motion management system and technology to deliver high dose of radiation therapy that has increased the usage and literature about radiation therapy in liver tumors regarding both response to treatment and toxicities. In liver tumors, radiation therapy is mostly recommended in hepatocellular carcinoma (HCC), intra-hepatic cholangiocarcinoma and liver metastasis.

The most significant radiation induced liver toxicity was described by Ingold et al. as "Radiation hepatitis" [1]. Historically, radiation to liver lesions with curative intent or incidental exposure during adjacent organ treatment or total body irradiation implied whole organ irradiation due to lack of high precision technology. This kind of whole organ irradiation led to a classic clinical picture which was then termed as "RILD." In 1966, Reed et al. have worked on pathology of radiation injury to liver and have established that the early changes are obliteration of small vasculature followed by secondary effects such as hyperemia and cell loss. They have also concluded that there is effective re-establishment of hepatic vasculature and return of normal hepatic structure with time [2]. Liver consists of hepatocytes connected as parallel structures and hence liver is considered a 'parallel' structure. This means, even if a small portion of liver is damaged, other part of the liver will work as 'parallel' structure and there will be no functional damage. If a large portion of liver is damaged and hence the 'parallel' architecture is affected then there will be disruption of function. This means, mean dose to liver is critical, whereas maximum dose or small high dose to liver may not have clinical relevance. In conventional fractionation, the whole liver could be treated only to the doses of 30–35Gy safely which serves only the purpose of palliation rather than cure. This aspect had set radiation aside of the curative liver therapy for many decades. With the advent of technological advancements like IMRT, especially SBRT, the notion of highly precise and accurate treatment has been made practically possible. This enabled focusing high doses of radiation to the tumor, sparing the normal liver thus bringing back the option of radiation for liver lesions into light once again. With the use of these, a significant portion of liver could be saved from high doses of radiation. The toxicity profile for this kind of focused radiation was certainly different from that of whole organ irradiation. There have been attempts made to characterize the effects caused by the high precision radiation. Thus the QUANTEC liver paper distinguished RILD to 'classic' and 'non-classic' types [3].

1.1 Classic RILD

Defined as 'anicteric hepatomegaly and ascites', also can also have elevated alkaline phosphatase (more than twice the upper limit of normal or baseline value).

This is the type of clinical picture encountered following irradiation of whole or greater part of the organ. As explained by Reed and Cox [2], this is related to the hepatic vascular changes leading to hepatic parenchymal necrosis. Although it takes time, this phenomenon is seen to be reversible in most of the cases. But the repair of hepatic structure is dependent on the baseline liver status. The incidence described in the 2000s was 5–10% if mean liver dose constraint of 30–35 Gy was met.

1.2 Non-classic RILD

Defined by elevated liver transaminases more than five times the upper limit of normal or a decline in liver function (measured by a worsening of Child-Pugh score by 2 or more), in the absence of classic RILD. In patients with baseline values more than five times the upper limit of normal, CTCAE Grade 4 levels within 3 months after completion of RT.

This is the type of RILD that is encountered typically after high dose radiation to a smaller part of liver. It is commonly associated with infective etiology. Although the exact pathogenesis is un-clear, it involves loss of regenerating hepatocytes. This is usually not irreversible.

The characteristics of them are summarized in **Table 1**.

2. Grade of toxicity

Common Terminology Criteria for Adverse Events (CTCAE) version 5 has graded various symptoms like hepatic pain, hepatic necrosis, hepatic hemorrhage distinctly. Hepatic failure is defined as a disorder characterized by the inability of the liver to metabolize chemicals in the body. Asterixis, mild encephalopathy is grade 3 whereas moderate to severe encephalopathy and coma is grade 4 and death is grade 5 (**Table 2**).

Taking into account the wider applicability in cancer treatment, the CTCAE toxicity grading is non-specific to radiation induced toxicity. It does not take into

	Classic RILD	Non-classic RILD
Time to presentation post Rx	2 weeks to 3 months	1 week to 3 months
Prone candidates	Otherwise fairly well-functioning pre-treatment liver	Common in those with poor liver function (hepatitis B infection, Child-Pugh Classes B and C)
Patho-physiology	There is occlusion and obliteration of the central veins of the hepatic lobules, retrograde congestion, and secondary hepatocyte necrosis	Un-clear but involves loss of regenerating hepatocytes and reactivation of hepatitis
Jaundice	–	++
Ascites	+++	+
Laboratory findings		
Increased Bilirubin	+	+++
Increased AST	2 times ULN	5 times ULN
Increased ALP	+++	+

Table 1.
Differences between classic and non-classic RILD.

consideration the performance status of the patient, baseline liver function and the relative changes in liver function caused by radiation, which is more clinically relevant and a predictor of reversibility of the RILD.

The Radiation Therapy Oncology Group (RTOG) liver toxicity grading includes nausea, dyspepsia as grade 1, abnormal liver function tests with normal serum albumin as grade 2, disabling hepatic insufficiency with low albumin, edema, ascites as grade 3 and necrosis, encephalopathy, hepatic coma as grade 4, death as grade 5 (**Table 3**) [4].

The drawback of this grading system is again the lack of specificity in scoring of liver function tests.

3. Time of RILD and presenting symptoms

RILD can be an acute or sub-acute phenomenon. It typically occurs 4–8 weeks, but can occur 7–90 days post radiation [5]. Rarely, it is seen to occur as late as 7 months. Though there has not been much variation in time to presentation between classic and non-classic RILD, classic tends to occur earlier. The clinical manifestations of RILD are non-specific but patients typically present with symptoms like fatigue, weight gain, increased abdominal girth, rarely abdominal pain. There can be signs of hepato-megaly, ascites, altered liver function, elevated alkaline phosphatase disproportionate to other liver enzymes. In case of non-classic RILD, there can be jaundice and marked elevation of liver enzymes. RILD is essentially a diagnosis of exclusion. Radiologic sequel is seen as sharply demarcated low attenuation areas on CT. In case of steatotac-tic liver background, there can be areas of elevated attenuation. MRI can show areas of increased T2 signal keeping in with acute inflammation [6].

CTCAE term	Grade 1	Grade 2	Grade 3	Grade 4
Hepatic pain (Sensation of marked discomfort in the liver region)	Mild pain	Moderate pain; limiting instrumental ADL	Severe pain; limiting self-care ADL	—
Hepatic hemorrhage (Bleeding from liver)	Mild symptoms; intervention not indicated	Moderate symptoms; intervention indicated	Transfusion indicated; invasive intervention indicated; hospitalization	Life-threatening consequences; urgent intervention indicated
Hepatic necrosis (A disorder characterized by a necrotic process occurring in the hepatic parenchyma)	—	—	—	Life-threatening consequences; urgent invasive intervention indicated
Hepatic failure (A disorder characterized by the inability of the liver to metabolize chemicals in the body)	—	—	Asterixis, mild encephalopathy; drug induced liver injury; limiting ADL	Life-threatening consequences; moderate to severe encephalopathy; coma
Sinusoidal obstruction syndrome (A disorder characterized by severe hepatic injury as a result of the blood vessels of the liver becoming inflamed and/or blocked)	—	Blood bilirubin 2–5 mg/dL; minor interventions required (i.e., blood product, diuretic, oxygen)	Blood bilirubin >5 mg/dL; coagulation modifier indicated (e.g., defibrotide); reversal of flow on ultrasound	Life-threatening consequences (e.g., ventilatory support, dialysis, plasmapheresis, peritoneal drainage)

Table 2.
CTCAE Grading of liver toxicity.

	Grade 0	Grade 1	Grade 2	Grade 3	Grade 4	Grade 5
Liver toxicity	None	Mild lassitude; nausea, dyspepsia; slightly abnormal liver function	Moderate symptoms; some abnormal liver function tests; serum albumin normal	Disabling hepatitic insufficiency; liver function tests grossly abnormal; low albumin; edema or ascites	Necrosis/ Hepatic coma or encephalopathy	Death directly related to radiation induced late effects

Table 3.
RTOG/EORTC late morbidity grading.

4. Evaluation parameters of radiation toxicity

Various empiric end points have been used to describe RILD, which include deterioration in Child Pugh score and RTOG/CTCAE grade 2–4 abnormal laboratory values. One such end point evaluated is Child Pugh (CP) score declining by 2 or more scores. Chapman et al. tried to define clinically relevant endpoints in cirrhotic patients post SBRT or proton beam therapy. In the retrospective review of 48 patients, multivariate analysis showed that Child Pugh Score increase of ≥1 or ≥ 2, CTCAE AST toxicity grade change were the strongest predictors of OS and RILD specific survival also [7]. This has been confirmed by other studies also. In a prospective study evaluating Child Pugh score as a tool for assessment of acute toxicity of liver SBRT, 94 patients were analyzed and 15% had RILD. In CP score assessment at 2 month follow up, 46 (38%) had no change in CP score. Decline of 1-, 2- & 3-point CP score from baseline was in 17%, 10%, 14%. Improvement in CP score of 1- & 2- point from baseline was in 9% and 1% respectively. CP score change after SBRT correlated with the post RT acute toxicities in the study and hence CP score change was considered as an objective scoring system to evaluate the radiation induced liver injury after SBRT treatment [8].

Other parameters include Model for End-stage Liver Disease (MELD) score, CLIP score, GRETCH score, albumin-bilirubin (ALBI) score, PIVKA, AFP grade (**Figure 1**).

4.1 MELD scoring system

The MELD score is a chronic liver disease severity scoring system that is calculated from serum bilirubin, creatinine and INR, but modified to include serum sodium concentration (MELD-Na) [9]. It was originally developed to predict three-month mortality following transjugular intrahepatic portosystemic shunt (TIPS) placement. It is frequently used for patients being evaluated for transplant.

4.2 CLIP scoring system

The CLIP score includes Child-Pugh stage, tumor morphology and extension, serum alfa-fetoprotein (AFP) levels, and portal vein thrombosis [10]. It takes into account both liver function and tumor characteristics and has been validated for HCC staging in relation to Okuda staging of HCC. But as a parameter for radiation induced liver toxicity, it is yet to be validated (**Table 4**).

4.3 ALBI score

ALBI score is a discriminatory method of assessing liver function in HCC with values of only albumin and bilirubin [11]. Validation of ALBI score as a tool in radiation

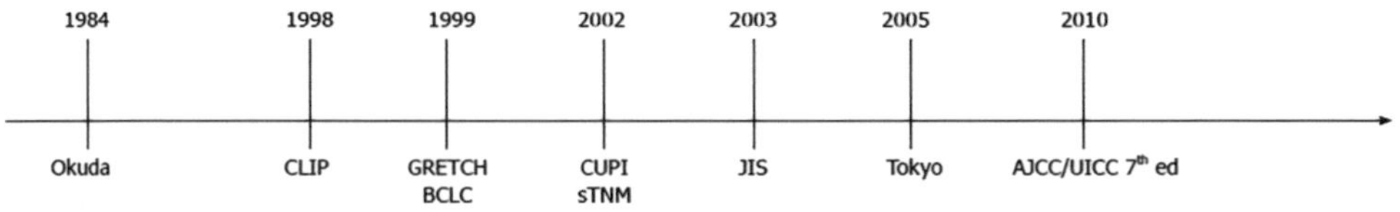

Figure 1.
Time frame of different scoring system.

	0	1	2
Child Pugh stage	A	B	C
Tumor morphology	Unimodular & extension <50%	Multinodular & extension <50%	Massive or extension >50%
AFP	<400	>400	
Portal vein thrombosis	–	+	

Table 4.
CLIP scoring system.

Weight	0	1	2	3
Karnofsky index	>80			<80
Serum Bilirubin (umol/L)	<50			>50
Serum ALP	<2x ULN		>2x ULN	
Serum AFP (ug/L)	<35		>35	
Portal obstruction	–		+	

Table 5.
GRETCH Scoring system.

toxicity assessment is undecided, but retrospective evidence indicates similar performance as with the CP score [12].

4.4 GRETCH score

The Groupe d'Etude et de Traitement du Carcinome Hépatocellulaire (GRETCH) score uses objective measures including bilirubin, alkaline phosphatase, AFP along with performance status and portal obstruction to predict survival outcomes. This prognostic system did not prove superior to other currently utilized scoring system and is not widely used world over [13] (**Table 5**).

4.5 AFP score

AFP is a well-established tumor marker for diagnosis of HCC that is detected in approximately 39–65% of HCC patients. AFP level normalization in a previously elevated patient within 3 months after SBRT is a prognostic surrogate for OS and PFS in patients with small HCC [14]. It is also useful in follow up of patients to detect early recurrence because the AFP level is related to the tumor activity. AFP stage for each prognostic group show clear survival differences ($P < 0.0001$), similar to the BCLC classification. However, survival differences among patient populations assigned to AFP stage B and C are not significant. In non-cirrhotic patients, the AFP staging system has a lower p-value than the BCLC classification.

4.6 PIVKA

Protein induced by vitamin K absence-II (PIVKA-II) is a potential screening marker for HCC and is an upcoming diagnostic tool that complements AFP [15]. Its role as a prognostic or predictive marker is yet to be determined.

Hepatocytes are involved in the synthesis of most coagulation factors, such as fibrinogen, prothrombin, factor V, VII, IX, X, XI, XII, as well as protein C, S, and antithrombin, whereas liver sinusoidal endothelial cells produce factor VIII and von Willebrand factor. Acute liver injury primarily decreases the vitamin K-dependent factors - prothrombin; factors VII, IX, and X.

5. Comparison between different evaluation systems

All these staging and scoring system have their own merits and demerits. Unfortunately, none of these scoring systems are validated in multiple prospective series. Hence, these systems are followed as per institutional preferences (**Figure 2** and **Table 6**).

6. Factors responsible for RILD

6.1 Radiation dose and RILD

Liver is a fairly radio-sensitive organ. This has been evident from the pain control rates of 73–83% have been reported after RT for HCC [16, 17]. In the 1991 Emami report, the liver tolerance doses or TD 5/5 (dose expected to result in 5% complication rate in 5 years) were set as 50 Gy for one-third of the liver, 35 Gy for two-thirds of the liver, and 30 Gy for the whole liver [18]. Nevertheless, the primary liver tumors have not been irradiated with curative intent for a long period of time attributed to the conventional radiation portals practically including the whole organ.

With the advent of SBRT, very high doses can be delivered focally to the tumor, which are known to result in vascular injury and also an ablative effect on the tumor,

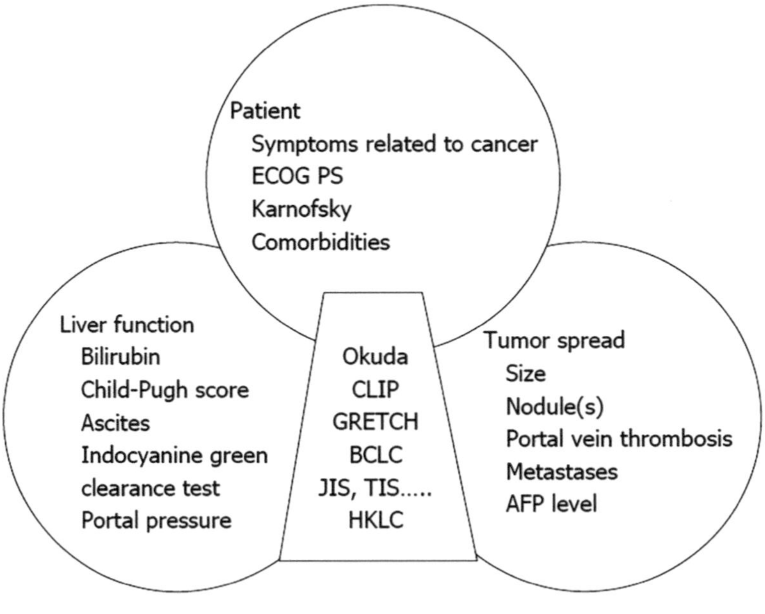

Figure 2.
Overlapping between different scoring systems.

	Okuda	CLIP	GRETCH
Child Pugh score		X	
Ascitis	X		
Albumin	X		
Total bilirubin	X		X
Alkaline phosphatase			X
Alpha fetoprotein		X	X
Tumor size	X	X	
Numbers of nodules		X	
Portal vein thrombosis		X	X
Presence symptoms			X

Table 6.
Comparison between different scoring systems.

in addition to the conventional DNA damage through dsDNA breaks. On the other hand, when these high doses of RT are being planned, one has to be extremely cautious regarding the precision and accuracy of the treatment. To account for inter and intra-fraction errors, various modalities like 4D CT, abdominal compression, voluntary breath hold, active breathing control and image-guidance during RT delivery can be used. The potential for tumoricidal doses to be delivered to focal HCC was first described by Dawson et al. at the University of Michigan by using an individualized dose allocation approach based on a normal tissue control probability (NTCP) calculation in 203 patients [19].

The Lyman–Kutcher–Burman (LKB)-NTCP model was used to assess dose-volume risk of RILD. The Lyman model assumes a sigmoid relationship between a dose of uniform radiation given to a volume of an organ and the chance of a complication occurring.

Various parameters have been looked into:

1. Effective volume (Veff): to allow volume-dose distribution comparisons between plans

2. TD50: tolerance dose associated with 50% chance of complication for uniform liver irradiation

3. m: steepness of dose response at TD50

4. n: defines the effect of the volume on a scale from zero to one [19].

Lausch et al. at the London Regional Cancer Program (LRCP), developed the logistic TCP model. They retrospectively reviewed 36 patients with HCC treated with median 4 Gy per fraction (range: 2–10 Gy) to a median cumulative dose of 52 Gy (range: 29–83 Gy) on a radiobiologically guided dose escalation protocol. The protocol called for prescribing the highest possible dose that met the constraint of keeping the estimated risk of RILD to <5%. They demonstrated that the D50 (dose that would result in a 50% LC) at 6 months was 53 Gy equivalent dose if given in 2 Gy fractions

(EQD2). In contrast, the D50 for metastatic disease to the liver was 70 Gy EQD2 demonstrating that HCC is relatively radiosensitive compared to other tumor types, including colorectal carcinoma metastatic to the liver. The D90 was found to be 84 Gy EQD2 suggesting that increasing dose results in increased LC [20]. Jang et al. developed another logistic TCP model based on tumor size. They demonstrated that higher doses (cumulative and per fraction) are required to achieve the same TCP for larger lesions. For lesions <5 cm vs. lesions >5 cm, doses had to be escalated from 51 to 61 Gy in three fractions to achieve a 2-year LC of 90%. They have also reported that D50 was 62.9 Gy EQD2 (range: 58–69 Gy EQD2) [21].

Ohri et al. published another TCP model from data of 431 primary liver tumors and 290 liver metastases. The 1-, 2-, and 3-year actuarial local control rates after SBRT for primary liver tumors were 93%, 89%, and 86%, respectively. Lower 1- (90%), 2- (79%), and 3-year (76%) actuarial local control rates were observed for liver metastases ($p = .011$). Among patients treated with SBRT for primary liver tumors, there was no evidence that local control is influenced by BED within the range of schedules used. For liver metastases, on the other hand, outcomes were significantly better for lesions treated with BEDs exceeding 100 Gy_{10} (3-year local control 93%) than for those treated with BEDs of ≤100 Gy_{10} (3-year local control 65%, $P < .001$) [22].

In 2010, Quantitative Analysis of Normal Tissue Effects in the Clinic (QUANTEC) reported recommendations that mean normal liver dose should be <18 Gy for baseline CP-A patients and < 6 Gy for those with CP-B, for a 6-fraction SBRT regimen (**Table** 7) [3, 28].

The dose recommendations for SBRT as per QUANTEC [3] for 5% or less risk of RILD are:

Mean normal liver dose (liver minus gross tumor volume).

<13 Gy for primary liver cancer, in three fractions.

<18 Gy for primary liver cancer, in six fractions.

<15 Gy for liver metastases, in three fractions.

<20 Gy for liver metastases, in six fractions.

<6 Gy for primary liver cancer, Child-Pugh B, in 4–6 Gy per fraction (for classic or non-classic RILD).

Critical volume model-based ≥700 mL of normal liver receives ≤15 Gy in three to five fractions.

6.2 Liver volume and RILD

Liver being comprised of hepatic lobules as functional subunits is a parallel organ. As a result, the mean dose and a critical volume being spared of high dose is of significance rather than the Dmax. The University of Colorado phase 1 clinical trial of SBRT for liver metastases described the importance of the liver volume spared, that is, the 'critical volume model,' a concept akin to surgical sparing of the future liver remnant. They have estimated that a typical normal liver volume is approximately 2000 mL and specified that a minimum volume of 700 mL or 35% of normal liver should remain uninjured by SBRT i.e. at least 700 mL of normal liver (entire liver minus cumulative GTV) had to receive at total dose less than 15 Gy [29]. This critical volume concept has also been applied to patients with HCC. Dyk et al. retrospectively analyzed 46 patients, of which 91% are CP-A status, treated with liver SBRT for either metastatic or primary liver malignancies and found the liver volume at 25 Gy (V25) > 32% was associated with CP-class progression on Univariate analysis [30].

Author	n	Selection	Dose	Radiation technique	Liver dose parameters	CP status (%)	Toxicity
Dawson et al. 2002 [19]	203	Unresectable intrahepatic cancer (HCC, cholangiocarcinoma, liver mets)	52.8 (range: 24–90)	3D-CRT	Median: 32.0 Gy (Range 14.9–44.0) LKB NTCP Median: 0.05 (Range 0.00–0.46)	—	RILD (n = 19, 9%) without RILD (n = 184, 91%)
Xi et al. 2013 [23]	41	HCC with marcovascular invasion	36 Gy (range, 30–48 Gy) in six fractions	SBRT using VMAT	Mean dose ≤18 Gy	Only CP class A	No Grade 4/5 toxicity
Andolino et al. 2011 [24]	60	HCC	CP A: 30–48/3 CP B: 24–48/5	SBRT	CP A: 1/3rd of the uninvolved liver was restricted to ≤10 Gy, and ≥ 500 cc of uninvolved liver received <7Gy. CP B: 1/3rd of the uninvolved liver was restricted to ≤18 Gy, and ≥ 500 cc of uninvolved liver received <12 Gy.	CP A: 36 CP B: 24	36.7%; 20% CP Progression 17 patients had grade 2 at baseline (out of 21 with grade ≥ 2 toxicity)
Tse et al. 2008 [25]	31	HCC and intrahepatic cholangiocarcinoma	36.0 Gy (24.0 to 54.0 Gy) in 6 fractions	SBRT	LKB – NTCP model	Only CP class A	Grade 3 liver enzymes were seen in five patients (12%).
Son et al. 2010 [26]	47	HCC	30–39 Gy (median: 36 Gy)	SBRT	V20 ≤ 50%; Total liver volume receiving <18 Gray (Gy) of radiation should be >800 cm^3	CP A: 89% CP B: 8% CP C: 3%	33% had ≥ Grade 2 hepatic toxicity 11% had progression of CP class
Mizumoto et al. 2012 [27]	259	HCC	66 GyE in 10 fractions to 77.0 GyE in 35 fractions	Proton Beam Therapy	Mean dose and V0–30 were identified as significant factors; preferred V0: 30%	CP A: 198 CP B: 58 CP C: 3	Change in CP score ≥ 2 in 11% at 12 months and 22% at 24 months

Table 7.
Summarizing various trials involving liver RT.

Son et al. retrospective review of 47 patients with HCC, of which 68% are CP-A status and showed the volume of normal liver receiving <18 Gy should be >800 cc to avoid CP class progression on Multivariate analysis [26]. Since all these studies constitute predominantly Child A patients, if these dosimetric parameters can be applied to Child B or C still uncertain. Indiana University group have further performed a phase II trial and reported their toxicity data in CP-A (n = 38) and -B (n = 21) patients [31]. For a treatment regimen of 48 Gy in 3 fractions, CP-A patients were required to either limit the dose to 33% of the uninvolved liver (D33%) < 10 Gy and/or maintain the liver volume receiving <7 Gy to <500 cc. For a more conservative treatment regimen of 40 Gy in 5 fractions, CP-B7 patients had to meet constraints of D33% < 18 Gy and/ or > 500 cc receiving <12 Gy. Dosimetric correlates were identified for grade 3 to 4 hepatic enzyme toxicity observed in 10.5% and 38.8% of CP-A and CP-B patients, respectively. However, the lower limit of the normal liver volume seems to vary between different races and ethnicities. Because heights and body weights vary so is the body surface area and so is the normal liver volume. Hence an absolute normal liver volume or its percentage to be spared may not be the optimal parameter to evaluate the liver function required for patients. The concept of body surface area (BSA) and Basal Metabolic Index (BMI) guided estimation of optimal liver volume need to be spared during SBRT treatment may be the future of liver SBRT program.

6.3 Type of radiation and RILD

The conventional techniques like 2D and 3D CRT led to more of classic RILD owing to the wide radiation portals. With the technological advancements like IMRT, robotic SBRT with tumor tracking high accuracy in radiation treatment became possible and the necessity for additional ITV margin has been eliminated. Sharp dose gradient helps to deliver higher dose to the target and spare normal liver. With real time image guidance high precision therapy, PTV margin can be cut down. Thus, high doses can be focused to the tumor with minimal margin. Although the incidence of RILD decreased, this may led to higher probability of non-classic RILD.

6.4 Co-morbidities and RILD

Cirrhosis: Background liver Cirrhosis plays a major role in development of toxicity. Cirrhotic patients are more prone to develop non-classic RILD than normal patients. Also, evaluation of the radiation induced changes turn out to be a tedious process because the baseline liver function would also have been abnormal. Radiologic differentiation between radiation induced changes and disease progression is also challenging.

Infective etiology: Infective etiology as such is not directly related to radiation induced toxicity, but again the background inflammatory picture and liver functional status play a role in diagnosis of RILD.

Re-irradiation: McDuff et al. analyzed 49 patients who received re-irradiation to liver. Mean interval from initial RT to first re-treatment was 411 days (range 61–1668 days). Mean BED2 (α/β = 10) were 76.93 and 77.60 for initial treatment and re-treatment, respectively. Mean BED2 (α/β = 10) were 76.93 and 77.60 for initial treatment and re-treatment, respectively. Only 1 patient (2%) met criteria for "non-classic" RILD demonstrating significant metabolic derangements in the absence of progressive disease. Another 6 patients exhibited metabolic derangements in the presence of progressive intrahepatic disease burden [32]. There have been case reports of safe and effective delivery of radiation to liver multiple times [33–36]. Appropriately selected patients under expert care can undergo re-irradiation in safety [37].

Nutritional status: Baseline nutritional status determines the general health of the patient and ability of the body to repair the radiation insult. Prior to the therapy, nutritional assessment thru hemoglobin, albumin, lactate dehydrogenase levels and the necessary corrections are recommended.

Disease stage: Disease status indirectly plays a role in development of toxicities. Larger the disease, larger will be the irradiated area and higher are the chances of RILD.

7. Re-irradiation in liver tumors

Re-radiation in liver tumors are not common in clinical practice. There are only few published literature in this aspect and no standard consensus regarding dosage schedule. In most of the subsites, such as in head & neck cancer or cervical cancer, in re-irradiation setting there is usually reduction of total dose (BED). Treatment volume is limited and fractionation schedule modified depending upon 'time to re-treat'. Irradiated volume also important in selection of fractionation schedule. Usually, in head & neck cancer 7 year time is considered 'safe' to re-challenge with full dose of radiation therapy. In case of re-radiation before that period, there is a reduction of dose depending upon the 'time to re-treat'. Usually 15% dose 'decay' considered in 1st year after radiation therapy and then every year 10% 'decay' in dose. As the time gap between primary radiation therapy and re-irradiation increase, safer to deliver higher (adequate) dose of radiation therapy to the target. In re-radiation of liver tumors this standard practice is not followed. In fact, in few studies there are better results (OS) in patients treated with higher dose in re-radiation setting. Child Pugh Score and 'time to re-treat' are considered significant prognostic factors. There is no compromise in irradiated volume as well. Tolerance of liver is low, but fortunately in re-radiation setting, liver tolerates radiation comparatively better than other subsites. High dose radiation therapy work like thrombo-embolism, embolizing blood supply to a portion of liver and stimulating proliferating of hepatocytes from adjacent normal liver. Proliferating hepatocytes causes hypertrophy of the liver portion which is naive to radiation therapy. This proliferating hepatocytes replace the post-CK necrotic liver. Hence, the 'new' regenerated portion of liver tolerate better than previously treated liver. Different cytokines liberated from the necrosed liver tissue may also stimulate hypertrophy of liver. After RT, there is fibrosis as well, and this fibrosis may lead to shrinkage of liver volume. Post-CK, there is 50% regression of the involved liver due to radiation injury, on the other hand there is 320% compensatory hypertrophy of the contralateral liver lobe [2]. This phenomenon negates the implications of firbosis, and hypertrophy has more predominant impact. Shrinkage of liver volume is expected to be more with higher integral dose of radiation therapy. In few studies, there is transient reduction of liver volume of about 20% at 3 months post-CK. However, at one year follow up there is only 10% shrinkage compared to pre-treatment volume. Even after repeat CK, liver volume is mostly maintained due to compensatory hypertrophy. Most severe complication after re-radiation is radiation induced liver disease (RILD). It is a syndrome of ascites, elevated transaminase level, and anicteric hepatomegaly. Usually occurs in a proportion of patient after receiving whole liver doses of >30–35 Gy. However, retrospective series of partial liver radiation have demonstrated that liver tolerance not only depends upon the total dose of radiation therapy, but also on pre-treatment Child-Pugh score, viral load and volume of tumor as well. Partial liver may be safely treated with radiation if adequate liver volume is preserved. In re-radiation, as the hypertrophied liver is mostly radiation naive, re-radiation is possible with adequate dose in small volume recurrences [33, 38].

8. Fiducial related toxicity

As stereotactic radiosurgery (SRS) applications moved to extra-cranial sites, the primary challenge was that SRS technologies were initially designed to deliver very precise treatments for non-moving targets. Therefore, methods to compensate for respiratory motion like fluoroscopy, surrogate markers [34] (spirometry, fiducials), 4D-CT and dynamic MRI were developed. Owing to the differential degree of movement of liver antero-posteriorly and cranio-caudally, and also between the lobes of liver, internal fiducial markers are ideal for tumor tracking. For fiducial tracking and CT slice thickness of 0.625 mm–1.25 mm, the system accuracy has been shown to be 0.7 +/− 0.3 mm. Per cutaneous fiducial insertion can be done ultrasonography guided or CT- guided under sterile conditions by interventional radiologist. Being an invasive procedure, complications like pain, bleeding, pneumothorax can be seen. Some of them might require chest tube placement, paracentesis, embolization. The technique of using "sterile blood patch" post fiducial insertion to prevent pneumothorax is in use. The main factor to prevent these remain the technical expertise. Apart from the acute complications, there can be migration of fiducials within the liver, rarely extra-hepatic sites also. Hence radiation planning and delivery is recommended to be scheduled after an interval of 48–72 hours post fiducial insertion [37, 39]. Park SH et al. retrospectively reviewed 101 patients with USG guided intrahepatic fiducial placement. There were no major complications, although 12 patients (12%) developed minor complications. Technical success was achieved in 291 (97%) fiducial placement. Of 101 patients, in 72/101 patients (71%) fiducials placement was ideal. Marsico M et al. (n = 15) assessed how different types of markers affects the tracking accuracy of Cyberknife. Ohta K et al. reported (n = 18) success rate of 100% (18/18) for fiducial placement in liver tumors. Only one patient (6%) had mild pneumothorax. There was no gross migration after placement. Choi J-H et al. (n = 32) evaluated the safety and technical feasibility of endoscopic ultrasonography (EUS)-guided fiducial placement. 23/32 patients (91%) had successful placement and only One patient (3%) developed mild pancreatitis which subsided with supportive care. Kim JH et al. (n = 77) evaluated the safety and technical success rate of an USG guided fiducial marker implantation. 21% had minor complications. Abdominal pain was the most common complication(14%). Fiducial migration occurred in 5 patients (6.5%). Dutta et al. analyzed 108 fiducials placed in 36 patients. Post-fiducial pain score 0–1 in 26 (72%) and score 3–4 was in 2 (6%). Five (14%) admitted in 'day-care' (2 mild pneumothorax, 3 pain). One patient (3%) admitted for hemothorax and died. Fiducial placement complications are usually rare, less than 3% patient need admission or have decompensation (change of Child Pugh Score > 2) [37, 39, 40].

9. Methods of prevention of RILD

The primary factor to prevent RILD is the better technique of radiation. SBRT with motion management techniques and real time tumor tracking is the best technique that can be used. Respecting the liver special constraints like mean liver dose and sparing a critical volume of liver from dose spill are the subsequent critical factors. Patient related factors like co-morbidities, nutritional status has to assessed prior to starting the treatment and the required dietary corrections have to be made. Feng et al. evaluated the role of amifostine as a radio protector in dose-escalated whole liver radiation therapy [41]. The study included 23 patients and a maximum dose of 40 Gy was used. This was compared with previously treated patients by logistical regression model. It was observed that the use of amifostine increased the liver tolerance by 3.3 +/−1.1 Gy. Selenium and Vitamin E are also shown to reduce the incidence of RILD in animal models by reducing liver lipid peroxidation and maintaining the endogenous liver antioxidant defense [34].

10. Management of RILD

No established therapies for classic RILD exist. There are no specific guidelines for the management of RILD. Suggestions for use of anticoagulants and steroids have been made, but it is primarily supportive care and diuretics are often used for the ascites. Although a few patients may recover, ample fraction will eventually die of liver failure. Thus proper patient selection to prevent RILD is crucial.

11. Conclusion

Radiation induced liver injury is potentially hazardous complication. There is no definitive treatment and a proportion of patient may land up in gross decompensation. Usually supportive care, diuretics, albumin supplement, vitamin K replacement may be useful. Better case selection will avert incidence of RILD. Precise imaging, contouring, planning and respecting normal tissue constraints are critical. Radiation delivery with motion management and image guidance will allow delivery of higher dose and spare normal liver and hence will improve response to treatment and reduce RILD.

Author details

Debnarayan Dutta* and Yarlagadda Sreenija
Department of Radiation Oncology, Amrita Institute of Medical Science, Kochi, Kerala, India

*Address all correspondence to: duttadeb07@gmail.com

References

[1] Ingold JA, Reed GB, Kaplan HS, Bagshaw MA. Radiation hepatitis. The American Journal of Roentgenology, Radium Therapy, and Nuclear Medicine. 1965;**93**:200-208

[2] Reed GB, Cox AJ. The human liver after radiation injury. A form of veno-occlusive disease. The American Journal of Pathology. 1966;**48**(4):597-611

[3] Pan CC, Kavanagh BD, Dawson LA, Li XA, Das SK, Miften M, et al. Radiation-associated liver injury. International Journal of Radiation Oncology. 2010;**76**(3 Supplement):S94-S100

[4] Cox JD, Stetz J, Pajak TF. Toxicity criteria of the Radiation Therapy Oncology Group (RTOG) and the European Organization for Research and Treatment of Cancer (EORTC). International Journal of Radiation Oncology, Biology, Physics. 1995;**31**(5):1341-1346

[5] Benson R, Madan R, Kilambi R, Chander S. Radiation induced liver disease: A clinical update. Journal of the Egyptian National Cancer Institute. 2016;**28**(1):7-11

[6] Maturen KE, Feng MU, Wasnik AP, Azar SF, Appelman HD, Francis IR, et al. Imaging effects of radiation therapy in the abdomen and pelvis: Evaluating "innocent bystander" tissues. Radiographics A Review Publication of the Radiological Society of North America Inc. 2013;**33**(2):599-619

[7] Chapman TR, Bowen SR, Schaub SK, Yeung RH, Kwan SW, Park JO, et al. Toward consensus reporting of radiation-induced liver toxicity in the treatment of primary liver malignancies: Defining clinically relevant endpoints. Practical Radiation Oncology. 2018;**8**(3):157-166

[8] Sreenija YKS, Nair H, Sasidharan A, Pottayil SG, et al. PO-1220 prospective evaluation of Child Pugh score as a tool for assessment of acute toxicity in liver SBRT. Radiotherapy and Oncology. 2021;**161**:S1010

[9] Malinchoc M, Kamath PS, Gordon FD, Peine CJ, Rank J, ter Borg PC. A model to predict poor survival in patients undergoing transjugular intrahepatic portosystemic shunts. Hepatology (Baltimore, MD). 2000;**31**(4):864-871

[10] A new prognostic system for hepatocellular carcinoma: A retrospective study of 435 patients: The Cancer of the Liver Italian Program (CLIP) investigators. Hepatology (Baltimore, MD). 1998;**28**(3):751-755

[11] Johnson PJ, Berhane S, Kagebayashi C, Satomura S, Teng M, Reeves HL, et al. Assessment of liver function in patients with hepatocellular carcinoma: A new evidence-based approach-the ALBI grade. Journal of Clinical Oncology: Official Journal of the American Society of Clinical Oncology. 2015;**33**(6):550-558

[12] Toesca DAS, Osmundson EC, von Eyben R, Shaffer JL, Koong AC, Chang DT. Assessment of hepatic function decline after stereotactic body radiation therapy for primary liver cancer. Practical Radiation Oncology. 2017;**7**(3):173-182

[13] Collette S, Bonnetain F, Paoletti X, Doffoel M, Bouché O, Raoul JL, et al. Prognosis of advanced hepatocellular carcinoma: Comparison of three staging systems in two French clinical trials. Annals of Oncology. 2008;**19**(6):1117-1126

[14] Jung J, Yoon SM, Han S, et al. Alpha-fetoprotein normalization as a prognostic

surrogate in small hepatocellular carcinoma after stereotactic body radiotherapy: A propensity score matching analysis. BMC Cancer. 2015;**15**:987

[15] Feng H, Li B, Li Z, Wei Q, Ren L. PIVKA-II serves as a potential biomarker that complements AFP for the diagnosis of hepatocellular carcinoma. BMC Cancer. 2021;**21**(1):401

[16] Kaizu T, Karasawa K, Tanaka Y, Matuda T, Kurosaki H, Tanaka S, et al. Radiotherapy for osseous metastases from hepatocellular carcinoma: A retrospective study of 57 patients. The American Journal of Gastroenterology. 1998;**93**(11):2167-2171

[17] Seong J, Koom WS, Park HC. Radiotherapy for painful bone metastases from hepatocellular carcinoma. Liver International. 2005;**25**(2):261-265

[18] Emami B, Lyman J, Brown A, Cola L, Goitein M, Munzenrider JE, et al. Tolerance of normal tissue to therapeutic irradiation. International Journal of Radiation Oncology. 1991;**21**(1):109-122

[19] Dawson LA, Normolle D, Balter JM, McGinn CJ, Lawrence TS, Ten Haken RK. Analysis of radiation-induced liver disease using the Lyman NTCP model. International Journal of Radiation Oncology. 2002;**53**(4):810-821

[20] Lausch A, Sinclair K, Lock M, Fisher B, Jensen N, Gaede S, et al. Determination and comparison of radiotherapy dose responses for hepatocellular carcinoma and metastatic colorectal liver tumours. The British Journal of Radiology. 2013;**86**(1027):20130147

[21] Jang WI, Kim M-S, Bae SH, Cho CK, Yoo HJ, Seo YS, et al. High-dose stereotactic body radiotherapy correlates increased local control and overall survival in patients with inoperable hepatocellular carcinoma. Radiation Oncology. 2013;**8**(1):250

[22] Ohri N, Tomé WA, Méndez Romero A, Miften M, Ten Haken RK, Dawson LA, et al. Local control after stereotactic body radiation therapy for liver tumors. International Journal of Radiation Oncology. 2021;**110**(1):188-195

[23] Xi M, Zhang L, Zhao L, Li Q-Q, Guo S-P, Feng Z-Z, et al. Effectiveness of stereotactic body radiotherapy for hepatocellular carcinoma with portal vein and/or inferior vena cava tumor thrombosis. PLoS One. 2013;**8**(5):e63864

[24] Andolino DL, Johnson CS, Maluccio M, Kwo P, Tector AJ, Zook J, et al. Stereotactic body radiotherapy for primary hepatocellular carcinoma. International Journal of Radiation Oncology, Biology, Physics. 2011;**81**(4):e447-e453

[25] Tse R, Hawkins M, Lockwood G, Kim J, Cummings B, Knox J, et al. Phase I study of individualized stereotactic body radiotherapy for hepatocellular carcinoma and intrahepatic cholangiocarcinoma. Journal of Clinical Oncology: Official Journal of the American Society of Clinical Oncology. 2008;**26**:657-664

[26] Son SH, Choi BO, Ryu MR, Kang YN, Jang JS, Bae SH, et al. Stereotactic body radiotherapy for patients with unresectable primary hepatocellular carcinoma: Dose-volumetric parameters predicting the hepatic complication. International Journal of Radiation Oncology. 2010;**78**(4):1073-1080

[27] Mizumoto M, Okumura T, Hashimoto T, Fukuda K, Oshiro Y, Fukumitsu N, et al. Evaluation of liver function after proton beam therapy for

hepatocellular carcinoma. International Journal of Radiation Oncology, Biology, Physics. 2012;**82**(3):e529-e535

[28] Munoz-Schuffenegger P, Ng S, Dawson LA. Radiation-induced liver toxicity. Seminars in Radiation Oncology. 2017 Oct 1;**27**(4):350-357

[29] Schefter TE, Kavanagh BD, Timmerman RD, Cardenes HR, Baron A, Gaspar LE. A phase I trial of stereotactic body radiation therapy (SBRT) for liver metastases. International Journal of Radiation Oncology. 2005;**62**(5):1371-1378

[30] Dyk P, Weiner A, Badiyan S, Myerson R, Parikh P, Olsen J. Effect of high-dose stereotactic body radiation therapy on liver function in the treatment of primary and metastatic liver malignancies using the Child-Pugh score classification system. Practical Radiation Oncology. 2015;**5**(3):176-182

[31] Lasley FD, Mannina EM, Johnson CS, Perkins SM, Althouse S, Maluccio M, et al. Treatment variables related to liver toxicity in patients with hepatocellular carcinoma, Child-Pugh class A and B enrolled in a phase 1-2 trial of stereotactic body radiation therapy. Practical Radiation Oncology. 2015;**5**(5):e443-e449

[32] McDuff S, Remillard K, Wo JY, Raldow A, Wolfgang JA, Hong TS. Safety and tolerability of liver re-irradiation. International Journal of Radiation Oncology, Biology, Physics. 2017;**99**(2):E171

[33] Dutta D, Krishnamoorthy S, Das R, Madhavan R, Nair H, Holla R. Third time re-irradiation of liver metastasis with robotic radiosurgery: A case series. Hepatoma Research. 2019;**5**:23

[34] Gençel O, Naziroglu M, Çelik Ö, Yalman K, Bayram D. Selenium and vitamin E modulates radiation-induced liver toxicity in pregnant and nonpregnant rat: Effects of colemanite and hematite shielding. Biological Trace Element Research. 2010;**135**(1):253-263

[35] Dutta D, Menon A, Abraham AG, Madhavan R, Nair H, Shalet PG, et al. Cholangiocarcinoma treatment with Synchrony-based robotic radiosurgery system: Tracking options. The Journal of Radiosurgery and SBRT. 2018;**5**(4):335-340

[36] Dutta D, Krishnamoorthy S, Sudahar H, Muthukumaran M, Ramkumar T, Govindraj J. Robotic radiosurgery treatment in liver tumors: Early experience from an Indian center. South Asian Journal of Cancer. 2018;**7**(3):175-182

[37] Dutta D, Tatineni T, Sreenija Y, Gupte A, Reddy SK, Madhavan R, et al. Hepatocellular carcinoma patients with portal vein thrombosis treated with robotic radiosurgery: Interim results of a prospective study. Indian Journal of Gastroenterology. 2021;**40**(4):389-401. DOI: 10.1007/s12664-021-01172-w

[38] Jose M, Pottikyal GS, Sasidharan A, Reddy SK, Haridas AE, Dutta D. Unusual presentation of an extrahepatic migration of a fiducial implanted for stereotactic body radiotherapy. Journal of Radiosurgery SBRT. 2021;**7**(3):257-260

[39] Dutta D, Kataki KJ, George S, Reddy SK, Sashidharan A, Kannan R, et al. Prospective evaluation of fiducial marker placement quality and toxicity in liver CyberKnife stereotactic body radiotherapy. Radiation Oncology Journal. 2020;**38**(4):253-261. DOI: 10.3857/roj.2020.00472

[40] Kataki K, Dutta D, Madhavan R, Kalita M. Prospective evaluation of migration, complications and utility

of fiducial placement for cyberknife treatment in hepatobiliary tumors. NJMR. 2020;**20**(1):10-15

[41] Feng M, Smith DE, Normolle DP, Knol JA, Pan CC, Ben-Josef E, et al. A Phase I clinical and pharmacology study using amifostine as a radioprotector in dose-escalated whole liver radiation therapy. International Journal of Radiation Oncology. 2012;**83**(5):1441-1447

Section 2

Disease-Related Hepatotoxicity

Chapter 5

COVID-19 Outcomes and Liver Disease

Umar Hayat, Hafiz Zubair, Muhammad Farhan, Ahmad Haris and Ali Siddiqui

Abstract

The novel severe acute respiratory syndrome coronavirus (SARS CoV-2) is the cause of coronavirus disease (COVID-19), a pandemic that represents a global health challenge. COVID-19 is usually a self-limiting disease; however, it is associated with a significant (3–7%) mortality rate. The excessive production of pro-inflammatory cytokines because of SARS-CoV-2 infection is mainly associated with high mortality due to multiple organ failure. The global burden of chronic liver disease (CLD) is vast. Approximately 122 million people worldwide have cirrhosis, 10 million living with decompensated cirrhosis. The preexisting chronic liver disease is associated with inflammation and immune dysfunction that might predispose to poor clinical outcomes in COVID-19, such as disease severity, rate of ICU admission, and mortality. The overlapping risk factors for SARS CoV-2 and chronic liver diseases such as obesity, advanced age, diabetes, and metabolic dysregulation are the major causes of these poor outcomes. Furthermore, progressive liver disease is associated with immune dysregulation, contributing to more severe COVID-19. This book chapter will explain the natural history and pathogenesis of COVID-19 in CLD patients along with the likely underlying SARS CoV-2-related liver injury mechanisms.

Keywords: SARS CoV-2, COVID-19, chronic liver disease, cirrhosis, hepatocellular carcinoma, COVID-19 clinical outcomes

1. Introduction

The severe acute respiratory syndrome coronavirus 2 (SARS-CoV-20) is a novel member of the coronavirus family first reported in Wuhan, China [1]. It causes COVID-19, which has infected millions of people worldwide, representing a global challenge. COVID-19 is generally a self-limiting disease presenting with flu-like symptoms but can also be deadly with a 0.7–5.8% fatality rate [2]. However, the disease severity and fatality vary by geographic areas and country, related to distinct population and disease demographics [2]. Mild COVID-19 cases may present with dry cough, fever, fatigue, dyspnea, and diarrhea. In contrast, severe cases may give a complex picture of acute hypoxia, respiratory distress syndrome (RDS), encephalopathy, and multiple organ failure [3]. Patients with advanced age and comorbidities such as hypertension, diabetes mellitus, obesity, chronic lung disease, chronic liver disease, cardiovascular disease, and cancer are at the greater risk of having severe illness and fatality due to COVID-19 [4]. Previously healthy patients with severe and critical COVID-19 also experience some liver injury, mainly presenting with deranged liver enzymes, such as aspartate aminotransferase (AST), alanine aminotransferase (ALT), and lactate dehydrogenase (LDH), and hypo-functioning of the liver in the form of hypoalbuminemia [3, 5–8].

COVID-19 leads to host immune dysregulation and cytokine storm by producing inflammatory markers [3]. This cytokine storm has been implicated in causing lung and liver injury and multiorgan failure (**Figure 2**). COVID-19 patients have been studied to have an elevated level of cytokines such as interleukin (IL)-1B, interleukin-6, tumor necrosis factor (TNF) interferon-gamma (INF-γ), interferon gamma-induced protein 10, macrophage inflammatory proteins (1alpha, 1beta), and vascular endothelial growth factor (VEGF) [3]. Although COVID-19 patients exhibit a highly variable immune response, the interleukin-6 level has been associated with COVID-19 severity and mortality [9].

The world is also dealing with another ongoing obesity pandemic due to sedentary lifestyles and food habitus [10]. This pandemic has led to various diseases such as diabetes mellitus, insulin resistance, and chronic liver disease (CLD) [10, 11]. CLD is prevalent worldwide and imposes a significant burden on healthcare costs and services. The most common causes of CLD include nonalcoholic fatty liver disease (NAFLD), alcoholic fatty liver disease (AFLD), viral hepatitis B and C. CLD can further progress to fibrosis, cirrhosis, and ultimately hepatocellular carcinoma (HCC) as an end-stage liver disease [10, 11]. Hepatocytes constitute a significant source of many proteins involved in both the body's innate and adaptive immune responses [12]. The liver plays a vital role in regulating immune homeostasis by two fundamental mechanisms. First, it prevents the systemic spread of dietary and microbial antigens from the gut; second, it produces the soluble molecules essential for effective body immune responses to the foreign antigens [12]. Thus, any liver injury can compromise the synthesis of proteins involved in the immune responses resulting in a compromised body immune surveillance against antigens [12]. It is categorized as an immune dysregulation in both CLD and liver cirrhosis.

The impairment of the liver's homeostasis in CLD leads to specific molecular patterns from the damaged hepatocytes, which may prompt the circulating immune cells to activate and induce an inflammatory response by releasing pro-inflammatory cytokines (interleukins and tumor necrosis factor) in the serum [13]. Furthermore, this immune dysregulation process emanates the possibility of increased infection susceptibility. Margot et al. have demonstrated that patients with CLD and cirrhosis are at a higher risk of morbidity and mortality due to COVID-19 infection [14]. However, the mechanisms of COVID-19-induced liver injury are multifactorial and are not fully understood [15, 16]. Cytokine storm hypothesis suggests that immune dysregulation because of SARS CoV-2 infections plays a vital role in liver pathophysiology in COVID-19 [15, 16].

This chapter aims to discuss the COVID-19 implications on healthy liver and CLD. The effect of COVID-19 on clinical outcomes in patients with cirrhosis and hepatocellular carcinoma will also be reviewed and discussed.

2. Pathophysiology of liver injury in COVID-9

SARS CoV-2 virus has two major binding sites. The spike glycoprotein (S) is essential for viral entry into the host cell, and the inner nucleocapsid phosphoprotein (N) interacts with the host RNA [17]. There are two possible mechanisms of liver injury in COVID-19 infection.

2.1 Viral immunological injury and systemic inflammatory response

One mechanism suggests that the SARS CoV-2 virus infects the target cells by binding to the angiotensin-converting enzymes 2 receptors on cell surfaces and replicates further inside to infect other cells [17]. These receptors are present on the bile duct epithelial cells, liver parenchymal cells, and alveolar type 2 cells in the lungs [18]. Some studies have suggested that the virus does not directly infect the hepatocytes, but it enters the portal circulation and, by reaching the liver, induces the Kupffer cells to activate immune systems, and thus produces inflammatory changes [19]. These inflammatory changes are the primary source of liver injury in SARS CoV-2 infection [19]. As a result of this inflammation, the liver enzymes (AST, ALT) were reported to be elevated >2 times the upper limit of normal in 14–53% of COVID-19 cases [20].

On the other hand, gamma-glutamyl transpeptidase (GGT) has been found to be elevated in 24% of the COVID-19 hospitalized patients suggesting a biliary epithelial cell injury [20]. Higher levels of liver enzymes have been associated with the severity of COVID-19 [21]. Moreover, antiviral drugs used for COVID-19 treatment are associated with liver injury. For instance, remdesivir use in severe COVID-19 patients has also been associated with elevated liver enzymes [22]. **Figure 1** illustrates the etiological factors of liver injury in COVID-19.

2.2 Hypoxic injury and cytokine storm

Hypoxia and cytokine storm following SARS CoV-2 infection can also affect the liver and are associated with multiorgan failure in some patients with severe COVID-19 (**Figure 2**) [23]. Hypoxia also causes Kupffer cells to produce more cytokines and triggers the recruitment and activation of other polymorphonuclear leukocytes to produce

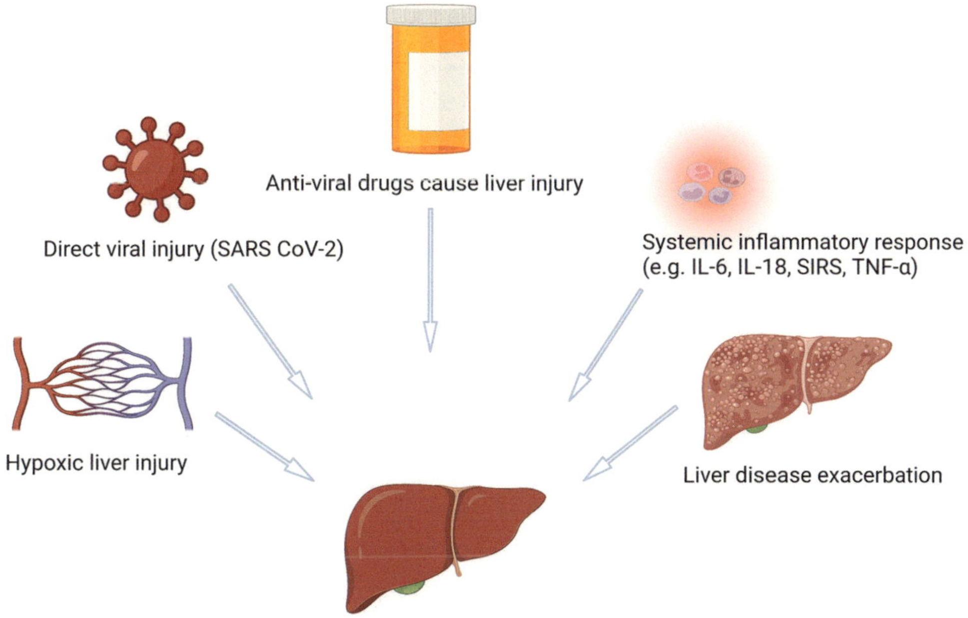

Figure 1.
Etiology of liver injury in COVID-19. Abbreviations: SIRS: Systemic inflammatory response syndrome; TNF-α: Tumor necrosis factor-alpha; IL18: Interleukin-18.

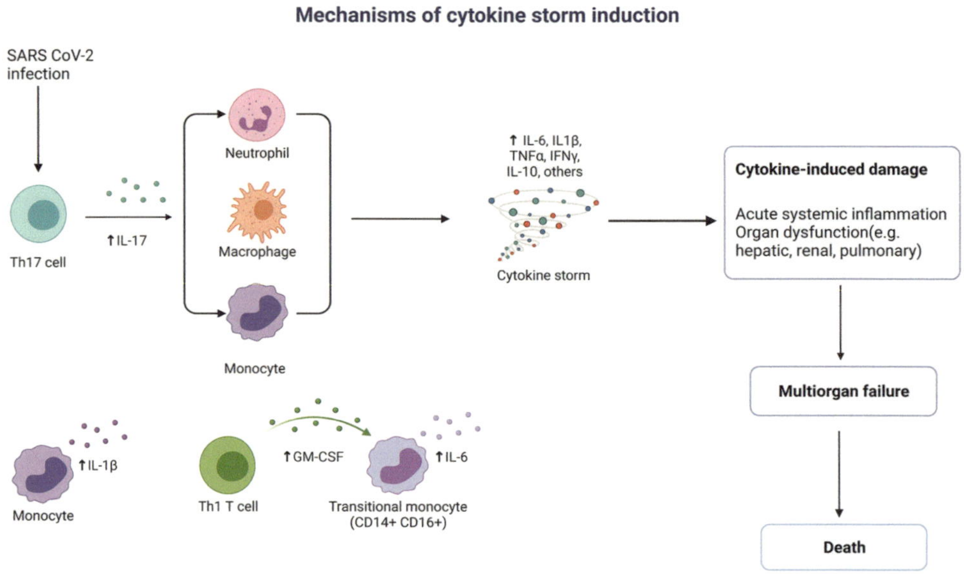

Figure 2.
Pathophysiology of SARS CoV-2 infection. A cytokine storm may occur following SARS CoV-2 infection, which can cause ineffective pathogen recognition with immune evasion leading to inappropriate inflammatory response or failure to return to the homeostasis mechanism.

more cytokines. This cytokine storm has also been implicated in thrombocytopenia and disseminated intravascular coagulation (DIC) observed in many COVID-19 patients [24]. Furthermore, it has been associated with liver vascular endotheliitis, complement system activation, and fibrin microthrombi formation in the liver sinusoids leading to hepatic dysfunction [25–28].

In essence, regardless of etiology, aminotransferases elevation is commonly observed in COVID-19 patients, and it appears to mirror disease severity [29]. Both ALT and AST have been observed to be elevated in 93% of hospitalized COVID-19 patients. However, most of the COVID-19 patients have been found to have AST predominant aminotransferase elevations. AST can be higher in non-hepatic injuries such as myositis, but correlations with creatinine kinase (CK) were weak [29].

3. Impact of COVID-19 on non-alcoholic fatty liver disease

Chronic diseases such as diabetes mellitus, hypertension, and obesity are associated with severe COVID-19 and lousy prognosis [30–33]. Together these conditions are part of the metabolic syndrome that predisposes to non-alcoholic fatty liver disease (NAFLD) [34]. The worldwide prevalence of NAFLD is 20–30% among Western populations and about 5–15% among Asian people. Thus, a large proportion of the population is at a higher risk of developing severe COVID-19 [35]. Shanghai et al. demonstrated that the patients with the fatty liver disease diagnosed on liver CT scan were more likely to have severe COVID-19 than the general population [36]. Elevated liver enzymes AST/ALT >2 times the upper limit are independently associated with the worst clinical COVID-19 outcomes [37–39]. Patients with NAFLD, compared with those without NAFLD, reportedly show a higher risk of liver enzymes elevation throughout the disease course (70% vs. 11.1%), a higher risk of disease progression (6.6% vs. 44.7%), and a longer viral shedding time (17.5 ± 5.2 days vs. 12.1 ± 4.4 days) [40].

The severity of liver fibrosis in NAFLD is associated with the worst COVID-19 clinical outcomes [41]. Furthermore, the patients with NAFLD who have been diagnosed with hepatic fibrosis on liver CT scan (OR, 4.32; 95% CI, 1.94–9.59) or with intermediate or high fibrosis index (Fib-4) (OR, 5.73; 95% CI, 1.84–17.9) have a significantly higher risk of developing severe COVID-19, regardless of the presence of other comorbidities [41, 42]. Moreover, the need for mechanical ventilation and ICU admission among COVID-19 patients was independently associated with diabetes mellitus, obesity, and FIB-4. FIB-4 is also associated with increased 30-day mortality (OR, 8.4; 95% CI, 2.23–31.7) [43].

It has been proposed that the patients with NAFLD/NASH have a higher expression of genes for ACE2 and TMPRSS2 receptors, which may explain the worse COVID-19 clinical outcomes among these patients. However, further studies are needed to support this hypothesis [44]. Because there is no therapy for NAFLD/NASH, it has been demonstrated that the patients with NAFLD/NASH are at a higher risk of COVID-19 severity, ICU admission, and mortality.

Similarly, metabolic-associated fatty liver disease (MAFLD) is one of the most common causes of chronic liver disease. It affects approximately 26–39% of the global population [45]. It is also a well-known risk factor for chronic diseases such as cardiovascular disease and diabetes mellitus, resulting in higher morbidity and mortality among these patients [45]. The criteria to diagnose MAFLD are based on hepatic steatosis and three other measures, including the presence of obesity, DM2, metabolic dysregulation [45]. Studies have demonstrated that preexisting MAFLD is linked with severe COVID-19 outcomes such as a high hospitalization rate and disease severity [46]. According to a proposed mechanism of liver injury in COVID-19 patients, the presence of MAFLD could release more pro-inflammatory cytokines to exacerbate the SARS CoV-2-induced inflammatory response [46]. SARS CoV-2 uses angiotensin-converting enzyme 2 (ACE2) receptors for cellular entry. The patients with MAFLD had reported having an increased expression of ACE 2 receptors, thus leading to more severe disease and worst clinical outcomes [47]. Lastly, MAFLD patients have an increased production of reactive oxygen species that further swirls the inflammatory storm responsible for disease severity [48].

4. COVID-19 and alcohol-associated liver disease

Worldwide alcohol consumption has been increased lately [49]. Social distancing and lockdown situations in the COVID-19 pandemic have further accelerated alcohol abuse, aggravating the alcohol-associated liver injury and chronic liver disease [50]. Alcohol consumption causes approximately 3.3 million annual deaths. CLD and cirrhosis are the main pathologies linked to alcohol consumption [50]. It has been suggested that excessive alcohol consumption may have immune-modulating effects in the human body and may predispose to bacterial and viral infections [51, 52]. Moreover, there has been an unprecedented rise in the listing rate for hepatic transplantation of ALD patients compared with HCV and NASH combined [53].

Patients with alcoholic liver disease (ALD) exhibit more severe liver injury if they have COVID-19 [14]. Therefore, ALD is independently associated with a 1.8-fold increased mortality risk among COVID-19 patients [14]. A recent study has indicated that alcoholic liver damage (OR, 7.05; 95% CI, 6.30–7.88) and alcoholic cirrhosis (OR,

7.00; 95% CI, 6.15–7.97) are significantly associated with the severity of COVID-19 [54]. Another study reported the higher severity of COVID-19 among patients with ALD. They have suggested this increase due to an increased proportion of alcoholic hepatitis among these patients due to a substantial increase in alcohol consumption since the pandemic's beginning [53, 54]. Future studies are needed to explore the mechanism and pathogenesis of how alcohol consumption and ALD are related to the severe COVID-19.

5. COVID-19 and liver cirrhosis

Cirrhosis is the end-stage of chronic liver disease characterized by advanced fibrosis. The liver is an essential part of the reticuloendothelial system and plays a vital role in immune regulation [13, 15]. It is responsible for innate immunity and responds to bacterial and viral infections. SARS CoV-2 binds to the selective ACE2 receptors on the surface of bile duct epithelial cells responsible for liver regeneration and immune response [50]. Thus, cirrhosis impairs this homeostasis response of the reticuloendothelial liver component and causes immune dysfunction leading to severe COVID-19 and a bad prognosis [54]. In severely decompensated liver cirrhosis, the pro-inflammatory state of the liver switches to the immune-deficient state [13].

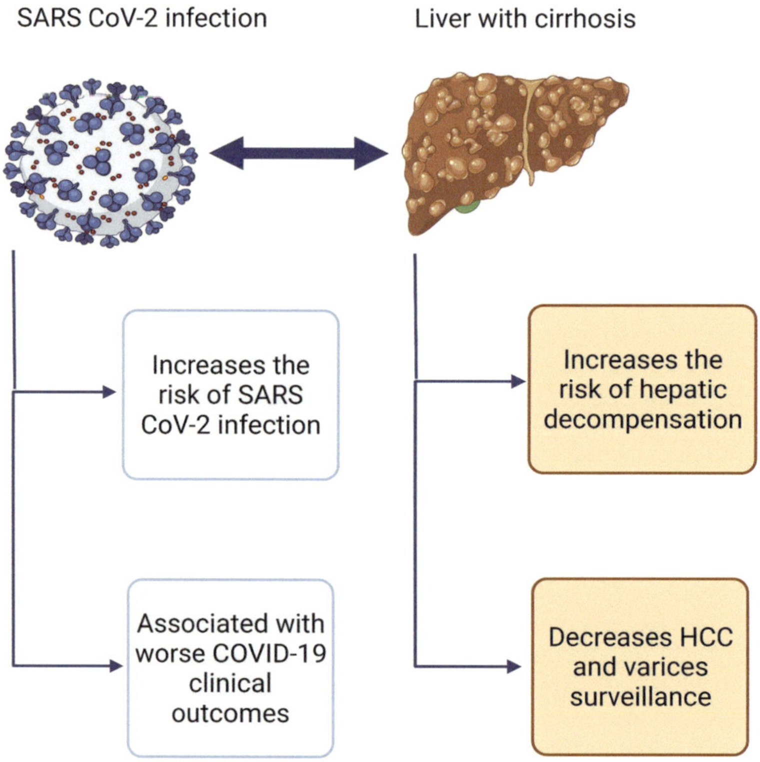

Figure 3.
COVID-19 and hepatic cirrhosis interrelationship. The impact of cirrhosis on SARS CoV-2 infection and vice versa.

Patients with cirrhosis are at an increased risk for SARS CoV-2 infection, a higher risk of developing severe disease, and a substantial risk for hepatic decompensation [55]. A large multicenter cohort study has demonstrated that COVID-19 infection was strongly associated with hepatic decompensation, increasing the mortality rate from 26.2% to 63.2% [56]. Moreover, studies have shown that cirrhosis is an independent predictor of overall and 30-day mortality in COVID-19 patients [57–59]. A recent analysis on 745 CLD patients infected with SARS CoV-2 virus in 28 countries indicated that cirrhosis was strongly associated with COVID-19 mortality (OR, 9.32; 95% CI, 4.80–18.08) [14]. Among the total, 150 patients died due to COVID-19, and among those, 123 had cirrhosis. The study also revealed that only 19% of the total deaths were due to cirrhosis-related complications, and for rest of the patients, the cause of death was lung injury [14]. These findings suggest that cirrhosis is a strong driving force for lung injury development in COVID-19 patients. This association is related to the cirrhosis-related immune dysfunction triggered by SARS CoV-2 infection [15]. Thus, the potential mechanism for severe COVID-19 in cirrhosis is the combination of cirrhosis-related immune dysfunction, an overwhelming systemic inflammatory response to SARS CoV-2 infection, and coagulopathy [60]. Lastly, cirrhotic patients have a poor response to Hepatitis B and pneumococcal vaccine, suggesting an inadequate response to SARS CoV-2 vaccination [61, 62]. The impact of cirrhosis on SARS CoV-2 infection and vice versa has been described in **Figure 3**.

6. COVID-19 and hepatocellular carcinoma

Hepatocellular carcinoma accounts for 6% of all the malignancies globally and is the sixth most common cancer [63]. Patients suffering from any malignancy are more prone to developing SARS CoV-2 infection and are at a higher risk of developing severe COVID-19 clinical outcomes [64]. Since SARS CoV-2 directly affects the liver parenchyma and leads to immune dysfunction, it can be hypothesized that the patients with HCC are more susceptible to the severity of the disease and have worse clinical outcomes than the patients with other cancers [65]. Moreover, cancer patients are more likely to be admitted to ICU and have mechanical ventilation and die (39%) than non-cancer patients (8%) [66]. A retrospective study on 28 cancer patients with two HCC patients has demonstrated that the patients with malignancies had poor outcomes compared with the general population [67]. It is also attributed to their advanced age, different comorbidities, and underlying cirrhosis. Also, these patients were more vulnerable to severe infection because of their compromised immunity resulting from poor nutrition status [67]. Additionally, recent chemotherapy treatment within the last month also increased the risk of COVID-19 severity [66].

AASL recommends restricting physician visits in this pandemic. They have also recommended continuing surveillance imaging for HCC with an acceptable delay of 2 months [68]. However, the management of these patients is becoming more and more challenging. It is expected that the interruption of the surveillance programs in high-risk patients and patients with cirrhosis will result in advanced HCC [65].

7. COVID-19 and viral hepatitis

Hepatitis B virus (HBV) and Hepatitis C (HCV) constitute two primary sources of chronic liver disease [69]. About 300 million and 70 million people are currently infected with HBV and HCV, respectively, instigating a significant burden to the healthcare system. HBV accounts for approximately 12%, and HCV constitutes about 11% of the underlying causes of chronic liver disease [69, 70]. The susceptibility of the HBV and HCV patients to get infected with SARS CoV-2 remains unclear. Similarly, there is only limited data available to conclude the association of HBV and HCV with the severity of COVID-19 [71]. Some studies have reported that viral hepatitis is not associated with the severity of the COVID-19 [72–74]. However, a small retrospective study has shown that COVID-19 patients with HBV disease had more severe disease e (46.7% vs. 24.1%) and a higher mortality rate (13.3% vs. 2.8%) than those without HBV disease [75]. The overall COVID-19 severity and mortality were found to be higher if the viral hepatitis patients have baseline liver injury and liver fibrosis than those without any liver injury (28.57% vs. 3.30%, P = 0.004) [76].

SARS CoV-2-induced lymphopenia and the use of immunosuppressive drugs such as corticosteroids may increase the risk of severe COVID-19 in patients with active or past HBV infection [76]. A retrospective study demonstrated that immunosuppressive therapy in COVID-19 has a low risk of HBV reactivation in patients with resolved HBV infection [77]. AASLD recommends continuing HBV and HCV treatment in COVID-19 patients if started before acquiring SARS CoV-2 infection [68].

8. COVID-19 and liver transplantation

Liver transplant patients are immune-compromised, thus vulnerable to SARS CoV-2 infection. It also makes them a potential source of infection dissemination to others, especially healthcare workers, by serving as super spreaders [78]. On the other hand, immunosuppression is considered protective against the severe COVID-19 infection as it suppresses the cytokine storm responsible for inflammatory changes [79]. Surprisingly, an international cohort study with 151 liver transplant recipients who had COVID-19 demonstrated that liver transplantation was not an independent predictor of mortality [80]. However, another study revealed that patients with liver transplants and COVID-19 had a higher mortality risk than those without transplantation (OR, 6.91; 95% CI, 1.68–28.48) [81]. COVID-Hep and SECURE-CIRRHOSIS registries described 159 liver transplant patients in their recent report. Of all, 81% were hospitalized, 30% were admitted to the ICU and required mechanical ventilation, and the overall mortality rate was 19% [82, 83]. The European Liver and Intestine Transplant Association (ELITA) revealed that the older patients with liver transplants had higher mortality [84]. In a systematic review of patients with solid organ transplants (SOT) who had COVID-19, the mortality rate among liver transplant recipients was 37.5% [85]. However, the risk of SARS CoV-2 infection and clinical outcomes of COVID-19 remained unclear among liver transplant patients and need further studies for factual inferences [86].

9. Conclusions

In essence, preexisting liver disease and liver injury are associated with the COVID-19 severity and mortality. The indicators of liver disease such as elevated liver enzymes, liver steatosis, and fibrosis are considered the prognostic markers of severe COVID-19. Additionally, CLD patients with severe COVID-19 tend to develop changes in fibrinolytic and coagulative pathways due to the dysfunctional innate immune response of the body against SARS CoV-2, leading to a lousy prognosis.

Moreover, the current co-occurring worldwide NAFLD/NASH pandemic is particularly relevant in the COVID-19 era as this mortal combination results in worse clinical outcomes. CLD patients should be given special attention for screening and treatment of COVID-19. Furthermore, patients with advanced liver disease and cirrhosis should be vaccinated on a priority basis. Lastly, the COVID-19 pandemic may have significantly delayed diagnosing and treating chronic liver disease and contributed to the significant morbidity and mortality associated with liver disease. Unhealthy behaviors and sedentary lifestyle changes in the pandemic can increase the global burden of liver disease in the future. Thus, the ongoing effect of the COVID-19 pandemic on the liver warrants robust measures and further investigation.

Conflict of interest

The authors declare no conflict of interest.

Author details

Umar Hayat[1*], Hafiz Zubair[2], Muhammad Farhan[3], Ahmad Haris[4] and Ali Siddiqui[5]

1 Department of Internal Medicine, University of Kansas, Wichita, Kansas, USA

2 Department of Internal Medicine, Creighton University Medical Center, Omaha, Nebraska, USA

3 Hospitalist Medicine, United Regional Hospital, Wichita Falls, Texas, USA

4 Hospitalist Medicine, Wesley Medical Center, Wichita, Kansas, USA

5 Division of Gastroenterology, Centura Healthcare, Rocky Vista State University, Denver, CO, USA

*Address all correspondence to: umarhayat216@gmail.com

References

[1] Zhu N, Zhang D, Wang W, et al. A novel coronavirus from patients with pneumonia in China, 2019. The New England Journal of Medicine. 2020;**382**:727-733. DOI: 10.1056/NEJMoa2001017

[2] Wu Z, McGoogan JM. Characteristics of and important lessons from the coronavirus disease 2019 (COVID-19) outbreak in China: Summary of a report of 72,314 cases from the Chinese Center for Disease Control and Prevention. JAMA. 2020;**323**:1239-1242. DOI: 10.1001/jama.2020.2648

[3] Huang C, Wang Y, Li X, et al. Clinical features of patients infected with 2019 novel coronavirus in Wuhan, China. Lancet. 2020;**395**:497-506. DOI: 10.1016/S0140-6736(20)30183-5

[4] Guan WJ, Ni ZY, Hu Y, Liang WH, Ou CQ, He JX, et al. China medical treatment expert Group for Covid-19. Clinical characteristics of coronavirus disease 2019 in China. The New England Journal of Medicine. 2020;**382**:1708-1720. DOI: 10.1056/NEJMoa2002032

[5] Li Y, Xiao S. Hepatic involvement in COVID-19 patients: Pathology, pathogenesis, and clinical implications [review]. Journal of Medical Virology. 2020;**92**:1-4. DOI: 10.1002/jmv.25973

[6] Hu LL, Wang WJ, Zhu QJ, Yang L. Novel coronavirus pneumonia-related liver injury: Etiological analysis and treatment strategy. Zhonghua Gan Zang Bing Za Zhi. 2020;**28**:97-99. DOI: 10.3760/cma.j.issn.1007-3418.2020.02.001

[7] Chen N, Zhou M, Dong X, Qu J, Gong F, Han Y, et al. Epidemiological and clinical characteristics of 99 cases of 2019 novel coronavirus pneumonia in Wuhan, China: A descriptive study. Lancet. 2020;**395**:507-513. DOI: 10.1016/S0140-6736(20)30211-7

[8] Shi H, Han X, Jiang N, Cao Y, Alwalid O, Gu J, et al. Radiological findings from 81 patients with COVID-19 pneumonia in Wuhan, China: A descriptive study. The Lancet Infectious Diseases. 2020;**20**:425-434. DOI: 10.1016/s1473-3099(20)30086-4

[9] Del Valle DM, Kim-Schulze S, Huang HH, Beckmann ND, Nirenberg S, Wang B, et al. An inflammatory cytokine signature predicts COVID-19 severity and survival. Nature Medicine. 2020;**26**:1636-1643. DOI: 10.1038/s41591-020-1051-9

[10] Sepanlou SG, Safiri S, Bisignano C, Ikuta KS, Merat S, Saberifiroozi M, et al. The global, regional, and national burden of cirrhosis by cause in 195 countries and territories, 1990-2017: A systematic analysis for the global burden of disease study 2017. The Lancet Gastroenterology & Hepatology. 2020;**5**:245-266. DOI: 10.1016/S2468-1253(19)30349-8

[11] Asrani SK, Devarbhavi H, Eaton J, Kamath PS. Burden of liver diseases in the world. Journal of Hepatology. 2019;**70**:151-171. DOI: 10.1016/j.jhep.2018.09.014

[12] Racanelli V, Rehermann B. The liver as an immunological organ. Hepatology. 2006;**43**:S54-S62. DOI: 10.1002/hep.21060

[13] Albillos A, Lario M, Álvarez-Mon M. Cirrhosis-associated immune dysfunction: Distinctive features and clinical relevance. Journal of Hepatology. 2014;**61**:1385-1396. DOI: 10.1016/j.jhep.2014.08.010

[14] Marjot T, Moon AM, Cook JA, Abd-Elsalam S, Aloman C, Armstrong MJ, et al. Outcomes following SARS-CoV-2 infection in patients with chronic liver disease: An international registry study. Journal of Hepatology. 2020;**74**:567-577. DOI: 10.1016/j.jhep.2020.09.024

[15] Fajgenbaum DC, June CH. Cytokine storm. The New England Journal of Medicine. 2020;**383**:2255-2273. DOI: 10.1056/NEJMra2026131

[16] Templin C, Ghadri JR, Diekmann J, Napp LC, Bataiosu DR, Jaguszewski M, et al. Clinical features and outcomes of Takotsubo (stress) cardiomyopathy. The New England Journal of Medicine. 2015;**373**:929-938. DOI: 10.1056/NEJMoa1406761

[17] Lan J, Ge J, Yu J, et al. Structure of the SARS-CoV-2 spike receptor-binding domain bound to the ACE2 receptor. Nature. 2020;**581**:215-220. DOI: 10.1038/s41586-020-2180-5

[18] Xu L, Liu J, Lu M, et al. Liver injury during highly pathogenic human coronavirus infections. Liver International. 2020;**40**:998-1004. DOI: 10.1111/liv.14435

[19] Chai X, Hu L, Zhang Y, et al. Specific ACE2 expression in cholangiocytes may cause liver damage after 2019-nCoV infection. BioRxiv. 2020.02.03.931766. DOI: 10.1101/2020.02.03.931766

[20] Bertolini A, van de Peppel IP, Bodewes FAJA, Moshage H, Fantin A, Farinati F, et al. Abnormal liver function tests in patients with COVID-19: Relevance and potential pathogenesis. Hepatology. 2020;**72**:1864-1872. DOI: 10.1002/hep.31480

[21] Cai Q, Huang D, Yu H, et al. COVID-19: Abnormal liver function tests. Journal of Hepatology. 2020;**73**:566-574. DOI: 10.1016/j.jhep.2020.04.006

[22] Grein J, Ohmagari N, Shin D, et al. Compassionate use of remdesivir for patients with severe COVID-19. The New England Journal of Medicine. 2020;**382**:2327-2336. DOI: 10.1056/NEJMoa2007016

[23] Wang H, Ma S. The cytokine storm and factors determining the sequence and severity of organ dysfunction in multiple organ dysfunction syndrome. The American Journal of Emergency Medicine. 2008;**26**:711-715. DOI: 10.1016/j.ajem.2007.10.031

[24] Sahu KK, Cerny J. A review on how to do hematology consults during COVID-19 pandemic. Blood Reviews. 2021;**47**:100777. DOI: 10.1016/j.blre.2020.100777

[25] Varga Z, Flammer AJ, Steiger P, Haberecker M, Andermatt R, Zinkernagel AS, et al. Endothelial cell infection and endotheliitis in COVID-19. Lancet. 2020;**395**:1417-1418. DOI: 10.1016/S0140-6736(20)30937-5

[26] Hooper JE, Padera RF, Dolhnikoff M, da Silva LFF, DuarteNeto AN, Kapp ME, et al. A postmortem portrait of the coronavirus disease 2019 (COVID-19) pandemic: A large multiinstitutional autopsy survey study. Archives of Pathology & Laboratory Medicine. 2021;**145**:529-535. DOI: 10.5858/arpa.2020-0786-SA

[27] Duarte-Neto AN, Monteiro RAA, Silva LFF, Malheiros DMAC, Oliveira EP, Theodoro-Filho J, et al. Pulmonary and systemic involvement in COVID-19 patients assessed with ultrasound-guided minimally invasive autopsy. Histopathology. 2020;**77**:186-197. DOI: 10.1111/his.14160

[28] Wang X, Sahu KK, Cerny J. Coagulopathy, endothelial dysfunction, thrombotic microangiopathy and complement activation: Potential role of complement system inhibition in COVID-19. Journal of Thrombosis and Thrombolysis. 2020;**15**:1-6. DOI: 10.1007/s11239-020-02297-z

[29] Bloom PP, Meyerowitz EA, Reinus Z, et al. Liver biochemistries in hospitalized patients with COVID-19. Hepatology. 2020;**73**:890-900. DOI: 10.1002/hep.31326

[30] Peng YD, Meng K, Guan HQ, et al. Clinical characteristics and outcomes of 112 cardiovascular disease patients infected by 2019-nCoV. Zhonghua Xin Xue Guan Bing Za Zhi. 2020;**48**:E004. DOI: 10.3760/cma.j.cn112148-20200220-00105

[31] Lighter J, Phillips M, Hochman S, et al. Obesity in patients younger than 60 years is a risk factor for Covid-19 hospital admission. Clinical Infectious Diseases. 2020;**71**:896-897. DOI: 10.1093/cid/ciaa415

[32] Zhou F, Yu T, Du R, et al. Clinical course and risk factors for mortality of adult inpatients with COVID-19 in Wuhan, China: A retrospective cohort study. Lancet. 2020;**395**:1054-1062. DOI: 10.1016/S0140-6736(20)30566-3

[33] Hill MA, Mantzoros C, Sowers JR. Commentary: COVID-19 in patients with diabetes. Metabolism. 2020;**107**:154217. DOI: 10.1016/j.metabol.2020.154217

[34] Portincasa P, Krawczyk M, Smyk W, et al. COVID-19 and nonalcoholic fatty liver disease: Two intersecting pandemics. European Journal of Clinical Investigation. 2020;**50**:e13338. DOI: 10.1111/eci.13338

[35] Satapathy SK, Sanyal AJ. Epidemiology and natural history of nonalcoholic fatty liver disease. Seminars in Liver Disease. 2015;**35**:221-235. DOI: 10.1055/s-0035-1562943

[36] Qian ZP, Mei X, Zhang YY, et al. Analysis of baseline liver biochemical parameters in 324 cases with novel coronavirus pneumonia in Shanghai area. Zhonghua Gan Zang Bing Za Zhi. 2020;**28**:229-233. DOI: 10.3760/cma.j.cn501113-20200229-00076

[37] Higuera-de la Tijera F, Servín-Caamaño A, Reyes-Herrera D, Flores-López A, Robiou-Vivero EJA, Martínez-Rivera F, et al. Impact of liver enzymes on SARS-CoV-2 infection and the severity of clinical course of COVID-19. Liver Res. 2021;**5**:21-27. DOI: 10.1016/j.livres.2021.01.001

[38] Khan A, Bilal M, Morrow V, Cooper G, Thakkar S, Singh S, et al. Impact of COVID-19 pandemic on gastrointestinal procedures and cancers in the United States. A multicenter research network study. Gastroenterology. 2021;**S0016-5085**(21):00460-00461. DOI: 10.1053/j.gastro.2021.02.055

[39] Shehab M, Alrashed F, Shuaibi S, Alajmi D, Barkun A. Gastroenterological and hepatic manifestations of patients with COVID-19, prevalence, mortality by country, and intensive care admission rate: Systematic review and meta-analysis. BMJ Open Gastroenterology. 2021;**8**:e000571. DOI: 10.1136/bmjgast-2020-000571

[40] Ji D, Qin E, Xu J, Zhang D, Cheng G, Wang Y, et al. Nonalcoholic fatty liver diseases in patients with COVID-19: A retrospective study. Journal of Hepatology. 2020;**73**:451-453. DOI: 10.1016/j.jhep.2020.03.044

[41] Targher G, Mantovani A, Byrne CD, Wang X-B, Yan H-D,

Sun Q-F, et al. Risk of severe illness from COVID-19 in patients with metabolic dysfunction-associated fatty liver disease and increased fibrosis scores. Gut. 2020;**69**:1545-1547. DOI: 10.1136/gutjnl-2020-321611

[42] Davidov-Derevynko Y, Ben Yakov G, Wieder A, Segal G, Naveh L, Orlova N, et al. The liver in severe acute respiratory syndrome coronavirus 2 (SARS-CoV-2) infection. European Journal of Gastroenterology & Hepatology. 2021;**33**:e313-e319. DOI: 10.1097/MEG.00000 00000002048

[43] Sterling RK, Oakes T, Gal TS, Stevens MP, deWit M, Sanyal AJ. The fibrosis-4 index is associated with need for mechanical ventilation and 30-day mortality in patients admitted with coronavirus disease 2019. The Journal of Infectious Diseases. 2020;**222**:1794-1797. DOI: 10.1093/infdis/jiaa550

[44] Meijnikman AS, Bruin S, Groen AK, Nieuwdorp M, Herrema H. Increased expression of key SARS-CoV-2 entry points in multiple tissues in individuals with NAFLD. Journal of Hepatology. 2021;**74**:748-749. DOI: 10.1016/j.jhep.2020.12.007

[45] Eslam M, Sanyal AJ, George J. International consensus panel. MAFLD: A consensus-driven proposed nomenclature for metabolic associated fatty liver disease. Gastroenterology. 2020;**158**(7):1999-2014. DOI: 10.1053/j.gastro.2019.11.312

[46] Sharma P, Kumar A. Metabolic dysfunction associated fatty liver disease increases risk of severe Covid-19. Diabetes and Metabolic Syndrome: Clinical Research and Reviews. 2020;**14**(5):825-827. DOI: 10.1016/j.dsx.2020.06.013

[47] Lefere S, Tacke F. Macrophages in obesity and non-alcoholic fatty liver disease: Crosstalk with metabolism. JHEP Rep. 2019;**1**(1):30-43. DOI: 10.1016/j.jhepr.2019.02.004

[48] Assante G, Williams R, Youngson NA. Is the increased risk for MAFLD patients to develop severe COVID-19 linked to perturbation of the gut-liver axis? Journal of Hepatology. 2021;**74**(2):487-488. DOI: 10.1016/j.jhep.2020.05.051

[49] WHO. GLOBAL Status Report on Noncommunicable Diseases. Available from: https://scholar.google.es/scholar?q=WHO.+GLOBAL+STATUS+REPORT+on+noncommunicable+diseases+2014.+n.d.&hl=es&as_sdt=0&asvis=1&oi=scholart. Accessed: 2014.

[50] Da BL, Im GY, Schiano TD. Coronavirus disease 2019 hangover: A rising tide of alcohol use disorder and alcohol-associated liver disease. Hepatology. 2020;**72**:1102-1108. DOI: 10.1002/hep.31307

[51] Pasala S, Barr T, Messaoudi I. Impact of alcohol abuse on the adaptive immune system. Alcohol Research: Current Reviews. 2015;**37**(2):185-197

[52] Szabo G, Saha B. Alcohol's effect on host defense. Alcohol Res Curr Rev. 2015;**37**:159-170

[53] Cholankeril G, Goli K, Rana A, Hernaez R, Podboy A, Jalal P, et al. Impact of COVID-19 pandemic on liver transplantation and alcohol-associated liver disease in the USA. Hepatology. 2021;**74**(6):3316-3329. DOI: 10.1002/hep.32067

[54] Wang QQ, Davis PB, Xu R. COVID-19 risk, disparities and outcomes in patients with chronic liver disease in the United States. EClinicalMedicine. 2021;**31**:100688. DOI: 10.1016/j.eclinm.2020.100688

[55] Banales JM, Huebert RC, Karlsen T, et al. Cholangiocyte pathobiology. Nature Reviews. Gastroenterology & Hepatology. 2019;**16**:269-281. DOI: 10.1038/s41575-019-0125-y

[56] Kushner T, Cafardi J. Chronic liver disease and COVID-19: Alcohol use disorder/alcohol-associated liver disease, nonalcoholic fatty liver disease/nonalcoholic steatohepatitis, autoimmune liver disease, and compensated cirrhosis. Clinics in Liver Disease. 2020;**15**:195-199. DOI: 10.1002/cld.974

[57] Moon AM, Webb GJ, Aloman C, et al. High mortality rates for SARS-CoV-2 infection in patients with pre-existing chronic liver disease and cirrhosis: Preliminary results from an international registry. Journal of Hepatology. 2020;**73**:705-708. DOI: 10.1016/j.jhep.2020.05.013

[58] Hashemi N, Viveiros K, Redd WD, et al. Impact of chronic liver disease on outcomes of hospitalized patients with COVID-19: A multicentre United States experience. Liver International. 2020 Oct;**40**(10):2515-2521. DOI: 10.1111/liv.14583

[59] Iavarone M, D'Ambrosio R, Soria A, et al. High rates of 30-day mortality in patients with cirrhosis and COVID-19. Journal of Hepatology. 2020;**73**(5):1063-1071. DOI: 10.1016/j.jhep.2020.06.001

[60] Marjot T, Webb GJ, Barritt AS, Moon AM, Stamataki Z, Wong VW, et al. COVID-19 and liver disease: Mechanistic and clinical perspectives. Nature Reviews. Gastroenterology & Hepatology. 2021;**10**:1-17. DOI: 10.1038/s41575-021-00426-4

[61] Aggeletopoulou I, Davoulou P, Konstantakis C, Thomopoulos K, Triantos C. Response to hepatitis B vaccination in patients with liver cirrhosis. Reviews in Medical Virology. 2017;**27**:e1942. DOI: 10.1002/rmv.1942

[62] McCashland TM, Preheim LC, Gentry-Nielsen MJ. Pneumococcal vaccine response in cirrhosis and liver transplantation. The Journal of Infectious Diseases. 2000;**181**:757-760. DOI: 10.1086/315245

[63] Tsamakis K, Gavriatopoulou M, Schizas D, et al. Oncology during the COVID-19 pandemic: Challenges, dilemmas and the psychosocial impact on cancer patients (review). Oncology Letters. 2020;**20**:441-447. DOI: 10.3892/ol.2020.11599

[64] Siegel RL, Miller KD, Jemal A. Cancer statistics, 2020. CA: Cancer J Clin. 2020;**70**:7-30. DOI: 10.3322/caac.21590

[65] Chan SL, Kudo M. Impacts of COVID-19 on liver cancers: During and after the pandemic. Liver Cancer. 2020;**9**:491-502. DOI: 10.1159/000510765

[66] Liang W, Guan W, Chen R, Wang W, Li J, Xu KE, et al. Cancer patients in SARS-CoV-2 infection: A nationwide analysis in China. The Lancet Oncology. 2020;**21**:335-337. DOI: 10.1016/S1470-2045(20)30096-6

[67] Zhang L, Zhu F, Xie L, et al. Clinical characteristics of COVID-19-infected cancer patients: A retrospective case study in three hospitals within Wuhan, China. Annals of Oncology. 2020;**31**:894-901. DOI: 10.1016/j.annonc.2020.03.296

[68] Iavarone M, Sangiovanni A, Carrafiello G, Rossi G, Lampertico P. Management of hepatocellular carcinoma in the time of COVID-19. Annals of Oncology. 2020;**31**(8):1084-1085. DOI: 10.1016/j.annonc.2020.04.007

[69] Tong S, Revill P. Overview of hepatitis B viral replication and genetic

variability. Journal of Hepatology. 2016;**64**:S4-S16. DOI: 10.1016/j.jhep.2016.01.027

[70] World Health Organization. Global Hepatitis Report. 2017. Available from: http://apps.who.int/iris/bitstream/10665/255016/1/9789241565455- eng.pdf?ua=1. Accessed: 2017.

[71] Lens S, Miquel M, Mateos-Muñoz B, García-Samaniego J, Forns X. SARS-CoV-2 in patients on antiviral HBV and HCV therapy in Spain. Journal of Hepatology. 2020;**73**:1262-1263. DOI: 10.1016/j.jhep.2020.07.007

[72] Zhang C, Shi L, Wang FS. Liver injury in COVID-19: Management and challenges. The Lancet Gastroenterology & Hepatology. 2020;**5**:428-430. DOI: 10.1016/S2468-1253(20)30057-1

[73] Liu R, Zhao LI, Cheng X, Han H, Li C, Li D, et al. Clinical characteristics of COVID-19 patients with hepatitis B virus infection—A retrospective study. Liver International. 2021;**41**:720-730. DOI: 10.1111/liv.14774

[74] Chen L, Huang S, Yang J, Cheng X, Shang Z, Lu H, et al. Clinical characteristics in patients with SARS-CoV-2/HBV co-infection. Journal of Viral Hepatitis. 2020;**27**:1504-1507. DOI: 10.1111/jvh.13362

[75] Chen X, Jiang Q, Ma Z, et al. Clinical characteristics hospitalized patients with SARS-Cov-2 and HBV Co-infection. Virol Sin. 2020 Dec;**35**(6):842-845. DOI: 10.1007/s12250-020-00276-5

[76] Zou X, Fang M, Li S, et al. Characteristics of liver function in patients with SARS-CoV-2 and chronic HBV co-infection. Clinical Gastroenterology and Hepatology. 2020;**19**:597-603. [Epub ahead of print]. DOI: 10.1016/j.cgh.2020.06.017

[77] Rodríguez-Tajes S, Miralpeix A, Costa J, López-Suñé E, Laguno M, Pocurull A, et al. Low risk of hepatitis B reactivation in patients with severe COVID-19 who receive immunosuppressive therapy. Journal of Viral Hepatitis. 2021;**28**:89-94. DOI: 10.1111/jvh.13410

[78] Saigal S, Gupta S, Sudhindran S, et al. Liver transplantation and COVID-19 (coronavirus) infection: Guidelines of the liver transplant Society of India (LTSI). Hepatology International. 2020;**14**:429-431. DOI: 10.1007/s12072-020-10041-1

[79] El Kassas M, Alboraie M, Al Balakosy A, et al. Liver transplantation in the era of COVID-19. Arab Journal of Gastroenterol. 2020;**21**:69-75. DOI: 10.1016/j.ajg.2020.04.019

[80] Webb GJ, Marjot T, Cook JA, Aloman C, Armstrong MJ, Brenner EJ, et al. Outcomes following SARS-CoV-2 infection in liver transplant recipients: An international registry study. The Lancet Gastroenterology & Hepatology. 2020;**5**:1008-1016. DOI: 10.1016/S2468-1253(20)30271-5

[81] Hammami MB, Garibaldi B, Shah P, et al. Clinical course of COVID-19 in a liver transplant recipient on hemodialysis and response to tocilizumab therapy: A case report. Am J Transpl. 2020;**20**:2254-2259. DOI: 10.1111/ajt.15985

[82] Moon AM, Baritt AS, Dhanasekaran R, et al. SECURE Cirrhosis Registry. Available from: https://covidcirrhosis.web.unc.edu/. Accessed: July 13, 2020

[83] Marjot T, Webb G, Cargill T, et al. COVID-Hep Registry. Available at: www.covid-hep.net/. Accessed: July 13, 2020.

[84] Belli LS, Duvoux C, Karam V, et al. COVID-19 in liver transplant recipients:

Preliminary data from the ELITA/ELTR registry. The Lancet Gastroenterology & Hepatology. 2020;**5**:724-725. DOI: 10.1016/S2468-1253(20)30183-7

[85] Nacif LS, Zanini LY, Waisberg DR, et al. COVID-19 in solid organ transplantation patients: A systematic review. Clinics (São Paulo, Brazil). 2020;**75**:e1983. DOI: 10.6061/clinics/2020/e1983

[86] D'Antiga L. Coronaviruses and immunosuppressed patients: The facts during the third epidemic. Liver Transplantation. 2020;**26**:832-834. DOI: 10.1002/lt.25756

Chapter 6

Non-Alcoholic Fatty Liver Disease and Its Potential Therapeutic Strategies

Youcai Tang, Xuecui Yin and Yuying Ma

Abstract

Non-alcoholic fatty liver disease (NAFLD) is diffuse steatosis of hepatocytes and is the most common type of chronic liver disease. The benign and reversible stage of NAFLD is defined as simple fatty liver, which further progresses to non-alcoholic steatohepatitis (NASH), liver fibrosis, and even liver cancer. It is believed that in the future, NASH would be one of the primary reasons for advanced liver failure and the need for liver transplantation. NAFLD is considered to be closely related to genetics, environment, metabolic diseases, such as obesity and hyperlipidemia. From the macro-level of NAFLD understanding, this chapter systematically analyzes the research progress on the etiology, pathogenesis, diagnosis, treatment, and development trends of NAFLD.

Keywords: non-alcoholic fatty liver disease, metabolic dysfunction-associated fatty liver disease, insulin resistance, type 2 diabetes mellitus, metabolic syndrome, gut flora, drug

1. Introduction

Non-alcoholic fatty liver disease (NAFLD) is a general term for a series of liver diseases ranging from hepatic steatosis alone (fatty liver) to non-alcoholic steatohepatitis (NASH), fibrosis, cirrhosis, and even hepatocellular carcinoma (HCC). Of these, hepatic steatosis alone (fatty liver) is known as NAFLD, and the occurrence of inflammation and liver cell damage is called NASH. Without effective intervention, the NASH may progress to cirrhosis. In the absence of alcohol or a small amount of alcohol, there is steatosis in more than 5% of liver cells, often combined with IR, metabolic syndrome (MetS), or type 2 diabetes mellitus (T2DM), and genetic variants of PNPLA3 or TM6SF2. The mechanisms are not fully understood but are involved in hepatic lipid accumulation, imbalance in energy metabolism, and inflammatory responses from various cell types. Lipid toxins, mitochondrial function, cytokines, and adipocytokines play major roles in a process of the disease. People with NAFLD often have insulin resistance, and a large number of T2DM patients develop NAFLD and its inflammatory complication NASH. The high incidence of NASH in patients with T2DM further leads to widely recognized complications such as cirrhosis and

HCC. There are no clear clinical criteria for the diagnosis of NAFLD due to the naming of an exclusive diagnosis and the emphasis on alcohol consumption, and ignoring the metabolic causes and heterogeneity of NAFLD. Therefore, in March 2020, an expert consensus from an international team consisting of 30 experts in 22 countries recommended changing the name of NAFLD to metabolic dysfunction-associated fatty liver disease (MAFLD) [1]. MAFLD is based on histological (liver biopsy), imaging, and blood biomarker to show the evidence of liver fat accumulation (hepatic steatosis), with one of the following three conditions: overweight/obesity, T2DM, and metabolic dysfunction. The prevalence of MAFLD is up to 25%, which poses a serious threat to human health and imposes a huge economic burden on society, and so far in the United States and the European Union, no drugs have been approved to treat this disease. Under the absence of proven and effective therapies, we must combine the etiology of NAFLD and its underlying pathological risk factors to explore therapeutic strategies.

2. Epidemiology

At present, the pathogenesis and potential pathological risk factors of NAFLD have not been concluded. The definition of NAFLD is also disputed, and these uncertainties prevent the large-scale diagnostic screening of NAFLD. However, the incidence of NAFLD is increasing year by year, and the age of onset is also decreasing through the Healthy People Census and related research reports. With the rapid change of lifestyle, the incidence of NAFLD is increasing year by year, and it has developed into a major global public health crisis. According to statistics, the prevalence of NAFLD is about 25% globally. The prevalence of NAFLD is approximately 24% in the North American general population, 32% in South America, 23.7% in the EU, and 27.4% in Asia [2]. In the past 10 years, the cases of fatty liver in China have jumped from 18% to 29.2%, and middle-aged men have become a high-risk population [3]. The incidence of NAFLD has increased with a rise in obesity, T2DM, and MetS, and according to 2016 statistics, the NAFLD patients in China are predicted to rise from 246 million to 315 million in 2030. Thus, if not controlled, the NAFLD will be one of the leading cause of cirrhosis requiring liver transplantation during the next decade. While the incline in the prevalence of NASH is from 2% to 3%, NASH has been recognized as the main cause of HCC and one of the indications for liver transplantation (LT) in the United States.

3. Etiology

Based on the pathogenesis, NAFLD can be divided into two types: primary and secondary [4]. Insulin resistance is related to genetic susceptibility, excessive weight gain, and overweight caused by excess nutrition, MetS-related fatty liver such as obesity, diabetes, hyperlipidemia, and cryptogenic fatty liver are all the primary causes. NAFLD caused by malnutrition, total parenteral nutrition, rapid weight loss after bariatric surgery, drug/environmental, industrial poisoning, etc. belong to the category of secondary group.

However, the new definition of MAFLD points out that hepatic steatosis is secondary, and should avoid using the terms "primary" and "secondary" fatty liver to describe. The previous dichotomous classification (simple fatty liver and NAFLD) was replaced by activity and fibrosis to better describe the process of MAFLD [1].

4. Risk factors

NAFLD is closely related to environmental and genetic risk factors, such as obesity, T2DM, MetS, lifestyle, genetic factors, and so on. It should be noted that lifestyle changes are strongly associated with the incidence of NAFLD.

4.1 Obesity

Obesity is recognized as an independent risk factor for NAFLD. The World Health Organization (WHO) defines normal as body mass index (BMI) 18.5 < BMI < 24.9, while it is defined as 18.5 < BMI < 23.9 in China. BMI has been the most useful population-level measurement for defining overweight and obesity, with equal or over 25 being overweight and equal or over 30 being obese. And the measurement applies to all adults of all ages. The Report on Nutrition and Chronic Disease Status of Chinese Residents (2020), which conducted a field investigation of more than 600,000 among nearly 600 million people in 31 provinces (autonomous regions and municipalities) across the country, found that more than half of the adult residents were overweight or obese. The overweight and obesity rates of children and adolescents aged 6–17 years old and under the age of 6 were 19% and 10.4%, respectively.

However, BMI neither reflects the distribution of body composition and fat, nor distinguishes between visceral fat and subcutaneous fat. For example, because muscle density is greater than fat, BMI will overestimate the degree of obesity in people with high muscle mass and underestimate the degree of obesity in people with high-fat contents. Therefore, although within the same BMI range, great differences exist in cardiovascular risk and mortality among individuals. Some overweight and obese people have normal metabolism and do not develop T2DM or dyslipidemia, and other metabolic diseases, which are known as metabolically healthy obesity [5]. On the contrary, part of the populations with normal weight has a variety of cardiovascular risk factors, which are prone to metabolic diseases such as T2DM, high blood pressure (HBP), and dyslipidemia.

Metabolic abnormalities are closely related to adipose tissue, mainly manifested as increased abdominal visceral fat [6]. Abdominal visceral fat is the deep adipose tissue wrapped by fascia, accounting for about 20% of the total fat mass in men and 5–8% in women. Compared with subcutaneous fat (SAT), abdominal visceral fat is more closely related to endothelial dysfunction. Glucose transporter-4 is highly expressed in abdominal visceral adipocytes, enhancing the rate of glucose uptake [7]. In addition, abdominal visceral fat is rich in β1, β2 adrenergic receptors, and unique β3 adrenergic receptors required for fat metabolism, so fats are broken down rapidly, producing more free fatty acids (FFA) and glycerol [8, 9]. FFA directly enters the liver through the portal vein, and excessive FFA deposition leads to the inhibition of hepatic glucose utilization, resulting in hepatic IR [10]. The increased oxidation of FFA in peripheral muscles will reduce the oxidative utilization of glucose in peripheral tissues, resulting in IR in peripheral tissues. The release of FFA into the blood will synthesize TG, resulting in TG deposition in many non-adipose tissues and organs.

Because of genetic background, lifestyle, and other reasons, Asian people show the characteristics of a thin body, less muscle content, and easy accumulation of abdominal fat. Under the same weight, they are more likely to develop a cardiovascular disease such as IR and glucose and lipid metabolism disorders than Caucasians. IR is the pathogenesis and core link of the normal-weight metabolic obesity [11]. Insulin can lower blood sugar mainly by inhibiting hepatic glucose production, stimulating the uptake of glucose by visceral tissues (such as the liver), and promoting the utilization of glucose by peripheral tissues (skeletal muscle, fat). IR refers to the decreased sensitivity of the target organs of insulin action (mainly liver, muscle, and adipose tissue) to the insulin action [12].

4.2 Type 2 diabetes mellitus

T2DM is characterized by relative insulin deficiency caused by pancreatic β-cell dysfunction and IR in target organs [13]. Globally, obesity, sedentary lifestyles, and aging populations have led to a marked increase in the incidence and prevalence of T2DM in recent years. As the sixth leading cause of disability in 2015, diabetes imposes considerable socioeconomic pressure on the public and significant costs on the global health economy. Long-term high blood glucose, large blood vessels, and micro blood vessels are damaged and endanger the heart, brain, kidneys, peripheral nerves, eyes, feet, and so on. According to the statistics of WHO, there are more than 100 complications related to diabetes. More than half of the deaths from diabetes are caused by cardiovascular and cerebrovascular diseases, and 10% are caused by nephropathy [14]. Amputations due to diabetes are 10–20 times as many as non-diabetic patients with diabetes. The mechanisms of microvascular and macrovascular complications caused by hyperglycemia are endothelial dysfunction, formation of advanced glycation end products, hypercoagulability, increased platelet reactivity, and high expression of sodium-glucose cotransporter-2 (SGLT-2) [15]. In addition, isolated postprandial hyperglycemia is more common in Asian diabetic patients. Unlike obese T2DM insulin resistance mechanisms, Asian non-obese T2DM had higher visceral fat. Although the BMI of Asian T2DM patients is lower than that of European and American T2DM patients, the visceral fat of Asian T2DM patients is higher than that of European and American T2DM patients. It has been studied that higher visceral fat is related to insulin resistance, which may be related to the lipolysis of visceral fat being higher than that of the subcutaneous fat [16]. The decomposed free fatty acids enter the liver through the hepatic portal vein, which increases triglycerides in liver cells and leads to insulin resistance. Defective β-cell function plays a key role in the pathogenesis of T2DM. In the presence of insulin resistance, if β cells can compensate by increasing insulin secretion, the body can maintain normal blood sugar; when the function of β cells cannot compensate for insulin resistance, T2DM occurs. IR results in increased lipolysis and ultimately more free fatty acids entering the liver. Reduced glycogen synthesis and increased gluconeogenesis in the liver are the main features of IR. In diabetic patients, abnormal lipid metabolism will easily lead to fatty liver, which in turn affects blood sugar control, resulting in a vicious circle, overall, fatty liver compromises the ability of hypoglycemic drugs to control blood glucose. IR is not only an important mechanism for the pathogenesis of diabetes but also attracts more and more attention to the central link of the pathogenesis of NAFLD. Previous studies have shown that fatty liver in diabetic patients is more likely to develop NASH, liver fibrosis, and cirrhosis than in non-diabetic patients. People with diabetes have a higher risk of developing fibrosis than non-diabetic individuals [17]. Currently, the histopathological biopsy is the only effective way to determine the presence and severity of NASH [18]. However, due to the limited understanding of NAFLD, NASH diagnosis in T2DM is often missed or diagnosed too late, resulting in the occurrence of end-stage liver diseases and serious consequences caused by metabolic disorders, such as cardiovascular and cerebrovascular diseases. The survival rates of patients also decline, while the medical cost will rise.

4.3 Metabolic syndrome

Metabolic syndrome (MetS) may have multiple causes, ranging from a set of unrelated risk factors to the series of risk factors linked by common underlying mechanisms [19]. Previously, MetS is often used as part of an overall risk assessment for cardiovascular disease. The diagnosis is based on abdominal obesity (highly associated with IR), decreased high-density lipoprotein cholesterol (HDL-C), elevated blood pressure, triglycerides, and fasting glucose (IFG or T2DM) [20]. The diagnostic criteria of the Diabetes Society of the Chinese Medical Association for MetS are adopted in China, and those who meet three or more criteria are MetS: a. BMI $\geq$ 25 kg/m^2; b. TG $\geq$ 1.7 mmoL and/or HDLC < 0.9 mmoL (male) or HDLC < 1.0mmo/L (female); c. SBP $\geq$ 140 mmHg and/or DBP $\geq$ 90 mmHg (1 mmHg = 0.1333 kPa) and/or diagnosed with hypertension and treated; d. FBG $\geq$ 6.1mmo and/or diagnosed with diabetic patients. NAFLD is considered as a hepatic manifestation of MetS. The liver, as a key organ of systemic metabolism, in turn, affects the risk of MetS and its complications. Increasing pieces of evidence show that the relationship between NAFLD and MetS are bidirectional [21]. These two clinicopathological syndromes share many aspects of their pathophysiology and IR is at the core of both. IR and MetS can exacerbate liver disease. Several cross-sectional studies have indicated that MetS and its components are associated with an increased risk of NAFLD in various populations compared with individuals without MetS.

4.4 Lifestyle

Rapid urbanization and lifestyle changes are associated with an increased incidence of NAFLD. Urbanization has led to an accelerated pace of life, dietary imbalances, such as irregular diets and high intake of saturated fat, carbohydrates, and trans-fatty acids, which are associated with IR and dyslipidemia. In addition, a sedentary lifestyle is also an important factor in NAFLD [22]. The fast-paced life and convenient transportation in cities make people less and less physically active in their daily and spare time. Age, increased smoking and alcohol consumption, screen time, decreased sleep, education, and stress all amplify the effects of IR and abdominal obesity, further increasing the prevalence of NAFLD.

4.5 Genetic factors

In addition to IR and MetS, genetic factors also play an important role in the occurrence and development of NAFLD. The human pastatin-like phospholipase domain containing 3 (PNPLA3) gene encodes 481 amino acid proteins called adiponutrin [23]. The exact role of this protein is still unknown, but it is thought to be a membrane-associated protein expressed in liver and adipose tissue, with lipogenic and lipolytic activities. It has been documented that it is located in lipid droplets (LDs) and may play a role in triglyceride hydrolysis. The gene is located in the long arm of chromosome 22. The variant rs738409 is the result of the substitution of cytosine by guanine, encoding isoleucine replaced by methionine at position 148 (I148M) of the protein. Substantial shreds of evidence suggest that this polymorphism is the strongest genetic determinant across the entire NAFLD lineage [23].

According to a study on the association of NAFLD among the medical patients in Uyghur and Beijing, it was found that the genotype frequency of PNPLA3-rs738409CG and GG genotype in NAFLD patients was higher than that in healthy controls, and the frequency of PNPLA3-rs738409G allele in NAFLD patients was higher than that in healthy controls [24, 25]. At the same time, the univariate logistic regression analysis of the genotype distribution of PNPLA3-rs738409 and NAFLD showed that compared with the PNPLA3-rs738409CC genotype, the GG genotype had a higher risk of NAFLD. Down-regulation of PNPLA3 mutant proteins will have beneficial effects on NAFLD and maybe a new therapeutic target for NAFLD treatment.

A similar situation was found in the transmembrane 6 superfamily member 2 (TM6SF2) gene. TM6SF2 is also present in LDs and mainly expressed in the liver and gut. It is believed as a key regulator of hepatic fat metabolism and secreting triglyceride-rich lipoproteins. The variant, identified as E167K, or rs58542926, is unrelated to NPLA3 variants but associated with susceptibility to NAFLD, and with advanced fibrosis and cirrhosis [26].

4.6 Gut flora

The influence of gut bacteria on liver homeostasis is based on an anatomical basis between the gastrointestinal tract and the liver, commonly referred to as the "gut-liver axis" [27]. The liver transports bile acids and antibacterial molecules (primary bile acids, IgA, and angiopoietin) to the intestinal lumen via the bile duct to control bacterial overgrowth and maintain intestinal flora balance. Liver products (bile acids) influence gut microbiota composition and barrier integrity. Under normal circumstances, intestinal mucosal epithelial cells, intercellular tight junctions, and biofilm constitute the mechanical barrier of the intestinal tract, which can effectively prevent harmful substances such as bacteria and endotoxins from entering the blood through the intestinal mucosa. Pathologically, microbiota-dysbiotic bacteria and their derivatives translocate to the liver through a disrupted gut barrier, where they cause hepatic inflammatory responses and commensal or metabolite-induced interactions that induce steatosis. In addition, there is increasing evidence that patients with NAFLD also have gut barrier dysfunction or altered gut permeability. Although the causal relationship between NAFLD/NASH co-occurrence and disruption of the gut epithelial barrier is unclear, impaired gut permeability exacerbates NASH [28].

5. Pathophysiology and pathogenesis

5.1 Theoretical hypothesis of "two-hit" and "multiple hit" in NAFLD

The pathogenesis of NAFLD is complex and still not fully clarified, and its pathogenesis was initially dominated by the"two-hit" hypothesis [29]. Hepatic steatosis is the first step in the development of NAFLD. A high energy intake from dietary fat, a marginal decrease in fatty acid oxidation, and an increase in hepatic lipid synthesis can all contribute to the abnormal accumulation of lipids in hepatocytes (the first hit). This process is associated with IR, which leads to dysfunction of intracellular triglyceride synthesis and transport. The "second hit" is based on the fact that lipid metabolism dysfunction and mitochondrial dysfunction occur in the liver, triggering inflammation and oxidative stress caused by fatty acid peroxidation mediated by cytokines, inflammatory factors, and endotoxins. These factors can trigger a series of signaling pathways, activate liver Kupffer cells, hepatic stellate cells (HSCs), immune cells, etc., and cause pathological changes in liver tissue such as inflammation, steatosis, and liver fibrosis to form NAFLD.

In recent years, as the public pays more and more attention to NAFLD, and the research on NAFLD continues to deepen and improve, the complexity of the pathogenesis of NAFLD is far more than the "two-hit" hypothesis, and the "multiple hit" hypothesis has emerged to explain it. The "multiple hit" hypothesis suggests that the progression of NAFLD involves the occurrence of "parallel, multiple" injuries [30]. Oxidative stress, lipid peroxidation, and IR, mitochondrial dysfunction, dysregulation of cytokines, activation of HSCs, and gut-derived bacterial endotoxemia caused by intestinal flora disturbance, as well as dietary habits, environmental factors, and genetic factors are in the occurrence and development of NAFLD play a role at the same time.

5.2 Insulin resistance

Insulin is a protein hormone secreted by pancreatic islet beta cells stimulated by endogenous or exogenous substances such as glucose and glucagon. The biological action of insulin at the cellular level is initiated by binding to specific receptors on the target cell membrane [31]. Insulin receptors are membrane glycoproteins composed of two separate insulin-binding domains (alpha subunits) and two signaling domains (beta subunits). The binding of insulin to the receptor causes conformational changes in α-subunit, so that adenosine triphosphate (ATP) can bind to the intracellular domain of β-subunit. After binding to ATP, the tyrosine kinase in the β- subunit is activated, which in turn auto-phosphorylates the insulin receptor [32]. Insulin mainly acts on the liver, muscle, and adipose tissue, and controls the metabolism and storage of the three major nutrients, protein, sugar, and fat. Normally, insulin reduces glucose production by reducing hepatic gluconeogenesis and glycogenolysis, accelerates glucose uptake by adipose and skeletal muscle tissue, regulates glucose homeostasis, and prevents the conversion of excess glucose to lipid deposition. Systemic or local IR occurs when the sensitivity and responsiveness of insulin target organs or tissues to endogenous or exogenous insulin are reduced. In a sense, IR is a compensatory response mechanism of the body to excess energy. Eating a lot of carbohydrates can cause our body to store more glycogen, which leads to the continuous release of insulin, the body's sensitivity to insulin slowly decreases over time, until eventually, maybe due to impaired insulin secretion, resistance to peripheral actions of insulin, or both. In IR, on the one hand, insulin cannot effectively promote glycogen synthesis, it specifically reduces hepatic gluconeogenesis and rapidly lowers blood sugar. On the other hand, it is the effect of lipid synthesis in the liver that leads to hyperglycemia and hypertriglyceridemia that greatly affects the metabolic balance of the body. IR in the liver is often associated with T2DM, MetS, and NAFLD [33].

5.3 Lipotoxicity

Adipose tissues play a central role in body metabolism by regulating fatty acid synthesis, release, and glucose utilization, maintaining the balance of skeletal muscle and liver metabolism. Therefore, fat accumulation is not only associated with obesity but also causes fat-related metabolic disorders, among which obesity-related IR is an important way to affect the body's energy stability. The original concept of lipotoxicity refers to the effect of excess FFA on the secretory function of pancreatic islet B cells under high-fat diet conditions [34]. With the deepening of research, it has been found that excessive lipid deposition in non-adipose tissues such as skeletal muscle, cardiac muscle, and liver can lead to cell dysfunction or cell death. Ectopic fat deposition leads to metabolic disorders of the corresponding organ, thus expanding the understanding of lipotoxicity. It is generally believed that excess intake of carbohydrates or fat gets stored in subcutaneous fat and visceral fat. When the storage capacity of adipose tissue is exceeded, especially in obese individuals, triglyceride from adipose tissue can be broken down to glycerol and FFA, and FFA can be mobilized by binding to plasma albumin. The FFA level in peripheral blood increases, an imbalance occurs in the uptake and metabolism of fatty acids. The utilization of FFA is hindered, resulting in insufficient lipid oxidation, thereby causing a large number of lipids and their products to accumulate in various tissues and organs. Inadequately oxidized lipids are stored in liver fat droplets in the form of triglycerides. Steatosis of the liver or fatty liver occurs when the accumulation of LDs in hepatocytes exceeds the storage and oxidative capacity of the liver. Steatosis of a large number of hepatocytes can induce liver dysfunction, including lipid accumulation and oxidative stress caused by lipid metabolites, inflammation, apoptosis, and liver fibrosis. This pathological process is called lipotoxicity. The failure of hepatocytes to deal with excess FFA-induced lipotoxicity promotes ER and oxidative stress leading to apoptosis, which is also a major feature of the NAFLD [28].

5.4 Endoplasmic reticulum stress

The endoplasmic reticulum (ER) is an organelle mainly responsible for physiological functions such as protein and lipid metabolism in eukaryotic cells. The membrane within the cytoplasm forms a series of sheet-like sacs and tubular lumens that communicate with each other to form a conduit system isolated from the cellular matrix. Because the conduit system is close to the inner side of the cytoplasm, it is called the endoplasmic reticulum. The ER is an important organelle related to metabolism. It has a sophisticated and complex control system to participate in intracellular anabolism and catabolism, such as protein synthesis and degradation, glycogen synthesis and decomposition, membrane lipid synthesis and recovery, fat storage, and hormone metabolism (such as production and secretion of insulin, leptin, resistin, etc.), and so on [35]. The ER is also a nutrient sensor in the body. Hyperglycemia, hyperlipidemia, and more inflammatory factors secreted by adipose tissue that accompany obesity are all stress signals of the ER. A long-term high-fat diet will increase blood sugar and fatty acids and induce disorder of glucose and lipid metabolism. Excessive high-sugar and high-fat substances entering cells for anabolism will increase the burden on the ER, increasing unfolded or misfolded proteins. When the accumulation of a large number of unfolded proteins exceeds a certain level, the corresponding unfolded protein response (UPR)-related signaling pathways are activated, resulting in an imbalance of ER function homeostasis. This state of homeostatic imbalance is called ER stress. The URP pathway is highly conserved and mainly mediated by three ER transmembrane proteins: pancreatic endoplasmic reticulum kinase (PERK), inositol-requiring enzyme 1α (IRE1α), and activating transcription factor (ATF6) [36]. It is generally believed that these three proteins all have domain located in the lumen of the ER, which can sense the concentration of misfolded proteins in the lumen. Under normal circumstances, ER stress inhibits the synthesis of nascent proteins, promotes the correct folding of unfolded proteins, and accelerates the degradation of misfolded proteins through its associated unfolded protein response (UPR) signaling pathway, thus exerting a protective effect on cells. However, once the UPR is activated excessively or persistently by ER stress, the endoplasmic reticulum-induced apoptosis pathway will be triggered, resulting in apoptosis. ER stress can also inhibit insulin signaling by activating UPR-corresponding kinases, such as IRE1α, phosphorylation of JNK, and IkB kinases [37]. In addition, related studies have also shown that FFAs-induced lipotoxicity also promotes ER stress and oxidative stress. CHOP (C/EBP-homologous protein), also known as GADD153 (growth arrest and DNA damage-inducible protein) or DDIT3 (DNA-damage inducible transcription 3). CHOP is considered a proapoptotic marker of ER stress-dependent cell death.

Elevated expression of the ER stress marker CHOP was detected in liver biopsies from patients with NAFLD [38], suggesting that ER stress-induced apoptosis in hepatocytes is likely related to the progression from steatosis to NAFLD in humans.

5.5 Inflammation

Although the pathogenesis of NAFLD has not been fully elucidated, the inflammatory response runs through the entire pathological process of NAFLD. In NAFLD patients, showing the increase of FFA released into the blood circulation and the decrease of the oxygen content of adipocytes, both act together to induce the activation of hypoxia-inducible factor (HIF1) and downstream target genes in adipocytes, and ER stress [39], resulting in cell death and specific inflammatory response. The inflammatory markers tumor necrosis factor-alpha (TNF-α), interleukin 6 (IL-6), and C-reactive protein (CRP) in NAFLD patients were significantly higher than those in healthy people [40]. TNF-α is secreted by macrophages and increases with the content of adipose tissues in the body. Highly expressed TNF-α induces phosphorylation and inactivation of insulin receptors in adipose tissues and smooth muscle cells, increases lipolysis to generate FFA, and inhibits adiponectin release. IL-6 is a cytokine produced by adipocytes and immune cells and has a complex regulatory mechanism in the body. The IL-6 production increases with the increased body fat and IR. It acts on the liver, bone marrow, and endothelium, increasing the expression of the acute phase reactant CRP in the liver. Several studies have shown a correlation between high CRP levels and the development of NAFLD as well [41]. Increased production and release of pro-inflammatory factors (TNF-α, IL-6, and CRP) can induce IR in the liver, skeletal muscle, and adipose tissue through insulin-interfering signaling pathways.

Therefore, inflammation and metabolic changes in adipose tissues can also trigger NAFLD.

5.6 Leptin and adiponectin

Adipokines also play an important role in the process of NAFLD-related liver fibrosis. Leptin is a hormone secreted by adipose tissue that can promote fibrosis [42]. The content of leptin in serum is positively correlated with the content of adipose tissue in the body. Normally, leptin functions primarily as an afferent signal in a feedback loop, acting on neurons in the hypothalamus to regulate feeding and other physiological functions. The researchers found that the level of leptin in the blood circulation increases when the body undergoes an inflammatory response, and many acute-phase factors, such as TNF-α, IL-1, IL-6, and bacterial lipopolysaccharide (LPS) stimulation, can rapidly increase leptin levels [43]. Leptin can also alter insulin action, induce angiogenesis, reduce endothelial NO synthase, and interact with the immune system [44]. In addition, leptin can activate HSCs by activating the JAK/STAT pathway. HSCs are the main source of extracellular matrix in liver fibrosis [45].

Adiponectin (ADPN) is also a protein hormone mainly secreted by adipocytes. ADPN mainly exists in blood circulation and plays an important role in the regulation of insulin sensitivity and glucose metabolism. ADPN reduces the level of plasma-free fatty acid (FFAs) by promoting fatty acid oxidation. There are two types of adiponectin receptors, adiponectin receptor 1 (AdipoR1) which is mainly distributed in skeletal muscle, and adiponectin receptor 2 (AdipoR2) which is abundantly expressed in the liver. Studies in mammals have shown that ADPN activates the adenylate-activated protein kinase (AMPK) signaling pathway through AdipoR1 and AdipoR2 [46]. Activated AMPK induces phosphorylation inactivation of acetyl-CoA carboxylase (ACC), thereby promoting fatty acid oxidation. In addition, peroxisome proliferator-activated receptor alpha (PPAR-α) is a key transcription factor regulating lipid metabolism in animals. As a downstream factor of the AMPK signaling pathway, it is also involved in the effect of ADPN on enhancing fatty acid oxidation [47]. Studies have shown that highly expressed ADPN attenuates the proliferation and migration of HSCs and promotes apoptosis of HSCs by inducing the expression of nitric oxide synthase (iNOS) and messenger RNA (mRNA) in HSCs, which hinders liver fibrosis [48]. In addition, blood ADPN concentrations are significantly reduced in MetS, diabetes, atherosclerosis, and NAFLD, in contrast to other cytokines, making ADPN a possible hallmark of these diseases.

5.7 Hepatic stellate cells

Hepatic stellate cells (HSCs) are a kind of non-parenchymal cells unique to the liver, accounting for about 8–13% of the total number of liver cells. HSCs have a dual phenotype of quiescence and activation [49]. In normal liver, the cells are quiescent. At this time, the cells act as hepatic fat-storing cells, and the intracellular LDs are abundant. The autofluorescence properties of vitamin-A stored in the LDs under the microscope contribute to the localization of the cells. During the development of NAFLD, multiple factors within the micro-circle promote the activation and transdifferentiation of HSCs into myofibroblasts. Activated HSCs can also massively secrete extracellular matrix (ECM), tissue inhibitors of metalloproteinases (TIMPS), matrix metalloproteinases (MMPs), and α-smooth muscle actin (α-SMA) [50]. The continuous activation of HSCs is a key link in the development and progression of liver fibrosis. On the one hand, HSCs produce 80% of type I collagen in fibrotic tissue, which induces liver remodeling. On the other hand, intra-hepatic sinusoidal pressure is increased by cell contraction. These two types of changes finally laid the pathological basis of NAFLD-related liver fibrosis. Existing studies have found that in the mechanism of liver fibrosis, growth factor signaling has a significant role in the activation of HSCs. Growth factors such as transforming growth factor (TGF)-α, epidermal growth factor (EGF), platelet-derived growth factor (PDGF), and other growth factors activate HSCs through signaling, promoting ECM remodeling, leading to collagen formation [51]. The molecular pathways of HSCs activation are complex and involve a variety of signaling pathways. The characteristics of HSCs and their roles in the repair of hepatocyte injury and local immunity in the liver still require more in-depth research.

6. Clinical manifestations

The onset of NAFLD is insidious, slow onset, and often asymptomatic. A small number of patients may have non-specific symptoms such as fatigue, mild discomfort in the right upper quadrant, dull pain in the liver area, or upper abdominal distension. With the development of the disease, some NAFLD patients may have symptoms such as jaundice, anorexia, nausea, and vomiting, which may be accompanied by hepatomegaly. In the decompensated stage of NAFLD-related liver cirrhosis, the clinical manifestations are similar to those of liver cirrhosis caused by other causes.

7. Diagnosis

NAFLD represents the liver manifestation of a multi-system disease, with heterogeneity in underlying causes, presentation, course, and outcomes. NAFLD means that the whole body is in a state of metabolic dysfunction.

Liver biopsy is considered to be the gold standard for defining NAFLD and able to distinguish steatosis from NASH. However, it is not recommended routinely because of the increased risk of bleeding and complications. Ultrasound is the most recommended and widely used diagnostic method for the identification of hepatic steatosis due to its sensitivity and non-invasiveness.

Over the past few decades, several expert groups have attempted to develop simple diagnostic criteria for clinical practice to identify NAFLD patients. The latest expert consensus in 2020 clarifies that the diagnosis of MAFLD is mainly based on histology, imaging, or blood biomarker evidence of the presence of fat accumulation in the liver (hepatic steatosis), in addition to one of three criteria (i.e., overweight/obesity, presence of T2DM or evidence of metabolic dysregulation) [1]. The presence of at least two metabolic risk abnormalities may correctly diagnose NAFLD in non-overweight/obese individuals.

8. Differential diagnosis

8.1 Alcoholic liver disease

Before the name of NAFLD was suggested to be changed to MAFLD, the difference between NAFLD and alcoholic liver disease (ALD) is mainly based on the prescribed amount and duration of drinking. Drinking history is a prerequisite for the diagnosis of ALD [52]. If there is no history of drinking, the diagnosis of ALD does not need to be considered. However, if the patient has a history of excessive drinking but the duration is less than 5 years or more than 5 years but the average drinking amount does not exceed the standard, this means that part of the population falls between the two diagnostic criteria when it comes to drinking.

After ethanol enters hepatocytes, it is oxidized by hepatic alcohol dehydrogenase, catalase, and hepatic microsomal alcohol oxidase, and finally forming acetaldehyde. Acetaldehyde has strong lipid peroxidation, and obvious toxic and side effects on hepatocytes, which hinders their metabolism and leads to degeneration and necrosis of hepatocytes. In addition, ethanol can affect the occurrence and development of liver disease by regulating intestinal flora, inflammatory response, and fibrosis [53]. Compared with NAFLD, patients with ALD have obvious liver disease presentation and rapid disease progression, and a higher risk of liver cirrhosis, liver failure, or liver cancer.

At present, a few studies have focused on the differential diagnosis of NAFLD and ALD, and many studies used non-fatty liver patients or healthy people as controls. There are still many problems and unknown factors in the differential diagnosis of NAFLD and alcoholic liver disease. Clinically, ALD is more likely to be diagnosed when there are obvious clinical manifestations of chronic hepatitis and cirrhosis, especially extrahepatic and neuropsychiatric manifestations. While NAFLD is more likely to be diagnosed when there are mild or even no symptoms. For the patients who drank alcohol, the changes of indicators within 4 weeks after abstinence were helpful for the differential diagnosis of NAFLD and ALD.

8.2 Chronic viral hepatitis

Viral hepatitis, as an infectious disease, is mainly caused by a variety of hepatitis viruses. There are five recognized types of viral hepatitis, namely hepatitis A virus (HAV), hepatitis B virus (HBV), hepatitis C virus (HCV), hepatitis D virus (HDV), and hepatitis E virus (HEV). All viral hepatitis is contagious, but the route of transmission and the intensity of infection vary. Hepatitis A and E are acute hepatitis, and types B, C, and D, are chronic hepatitis and can develop liver cirrhosis and HCC. Hepatitis D virus can only be transmitted in individuals with the presence of hepatitis B virus, so normal people do not get hepatitis D. Chronic viral hepatitis is an inflammation of the liver caused by the hepatitis virus that lasts for more than 6 months. The hepatitis virus usually causes symptoms after it has severely damaged the liver [54]. Viral hepatitis is an infectious disease with the highest infection rate and the greatest harm to patients in China.

HBV is an enveloped partially double-stranded DNA virus, consisting of an outer lipid envelope embedded with hepatitis B surface antigen (HBsAg) and a nucleocapsid containing hepatitis B core antigen (HBcAg), viral polymerase, and DNA genome. Clinically, it is difficult to distinguish hepatitis B from hepatitis caused by other viral agents, and the diagnosis must be confirmed by laboratory tests. The laboratory tests for hepatitis B surface antigen (HBsAg) are used to diagnose hepatitis B infection. Acute HBV infection is characterized by the presence of hepatitis B surface antigen-antibody and immunoglobulin IgM type anti-core antigen-antibody. In the early stage of infection, the serum of patients can also be positive for hepatitis B-e antigen (HBeAg). Chronic infection is characterized by the persistence of HBsAg-antibodies (with or without HBeAg positivity) (>6 months). The persistence of HBsAg-antibodies is a primary risk marker for the development of chronic liver disease and progression to HCC. The presence of HBeAg positivity indicates that the blood and body fluids of infected individuals are highly contagious [55].

HCV is a single-stranded RNA virus that can be divided into six genotypes and several subtypes. The genome of HCV encodes a single polyprotein that can be translated and processed into structural and nonstructural proteins. And the nonstructural proteins have key functions in viral replication. During the acute phase of HCV infection, the presence of an HCV-specific CD4-T cells response is associated with the control of viral replication. If the response of the CD4-T cell is sustained and maintained, HCV is permanently eliminated. If the CD4-T cells' response is lost, rebound viral replication or viremia occurs, resulting in a viral persistence [56]. In chronic HCV infection, CD4-T cells are functionally limited due to impaired proliferative capacity, which is caused by HCV core-mediated inhibition of IL-2 secretion.

8.3 Autoimmune liver diseases

Autoimmune liver diseases (ALDs) refer to a group of non-infectious liver diseases characterized by liver pathological damage and abnormal liver function. Its pathogenesis may be related to autoimmunity, mainly including autoimmune hepatitis (AIH), primary biliary cirrhosis (PBC), primary sclerosing cholangitis (PSC), and any overlapping syndrome of these three diseases. AIH is mainly causing damage to liver cells, while PBC and PSC are mainly damaging the biliary tract. The main damage is related to abnormal autoimmune function. ALDs are chronic diseases with a long natural history and progressive development, which eventually leads to liver cirrhosis and liver failure [57]. China still lacks exact statistics, but the number of clinically detected and reported cases has significantly increased in recent years. At present, it is believed that ALDs are caused by the breakdown of the immune system's immune tolerance to self-antigens, which induces an immune attack on the liver. Genetic susceptibility and environmental factors are the initiating factors, and the pathogenesis may be related to factors such as infection, chemical factors, cytokine networks, and molecular mimicry of self-antigens. However, the specific etiology and pathogenesis are still unclear, and there is currently no single clinical or laboratory index to diagnose ALDs. It is necessary to comprehensively integrate clinical manifestations, laboratory examinations, and liver histological characteristics to exclude other possible causes of chronic hepatitis. Clinically, patients with ALDs lack specificity. Initially, symptoms such as fatigue, pruritus, jaundice, and abdominal pain are often present. Biochemical tests are often abnormal in liver function. The presence of autoantibodies in serum is an important feature for diagnosis and differential diagnosis, such as ANA, SMA, AMAM2, etc., and histopathological examination of the liver is also very important [58].

8.4 Hepatolenticular degeneration

Hepatolenticular degeneration, also known as Wilson disease (WD), is an autosomal recessive genetic disorder caused by the mutation of the ATPase copper transport β gene ATP7B, resulting in disturbance of copper metabolism in the body [59]. The genetic mutations lead to the defective or loss of ATPase function, resulting in the obstruction of copper excretion in the bile duct, and a large amount of copper accumulates in the brain, liver, kidney, bone, joint, cornea, and other tissues or organs. The carrier frequency and prevalence rate of this disease in the world are 1:100–1:90, and 1:40,000–1:30,000 respectively. Clinically, the clinical manifestations of WD patients are diverse, and the clinical manifestations can be mainly divided into brain type, liver type, mixed type, and other types. The manifestations of cerebral-type patients mainly include Parkinson's syndrome, dyskinesia, oral and mandibular dystonia, and psychiatric symptoms. The main clinical symptoms of liver patients include asymptomatic elevation of transhelicase, hepatomegaly, splenomegaly, hepatitis, fatty liver, cirrhosis, and acute liver failure. Excessive copper will also be deposited in the kidneys, bones and joints, blood, skin, cornea, and other tissues or organs, causing corresponding tissue and organ damage. Since the human body's copper is mainly excreted from the liver in the form of bile, many liver diseases themselves can lead to abnormal copper metabolism indicators in the human body. Therefore, for patients with only liver involvement, the interpretation of auxiliary examination indicators needs to be more cautious, and a comprehensive evaluation should be combined with a variety of examination methods. The new 2021 health guidelines in China remind clinicians to be highly alert the individuals with serum ceruloplasmin <120 mg and children with elevated liver enzymes and 24 h urinary copper ≥ 40 μg. It is recommended to perform ATP7B gene testing to confirm the diagnosis.

Specific diseases, such as alcoholic liver disease, chronic viral hepatitis, autoimmune liver disease, and Wilson's disease that can lead to fatty liver need to be excluded, as well as drugs (tamoxifen, amiodarone, methotrexate, glucocorticoids, etc.), total parenteral nutrition, inflammatory bowel disease, hypothyroidism, Cushing's syndrome, lack of β-lipoproteinemia, and congenital IR syndrome-related fatty liver also need to be excluded.

9. Treatment

Generally, non-alcoholic fatty liver (NAFL) progresses relatively slowly. But when NAFL progresses to NASH without effective intervention, 15–25% of patients can progress to liver cirrhosis or even HCC within 10–15 years. Exploring and eliminating the causes are the fundamental ways to treat this disease. Obese people need to more effectively control their weight, and diabetic patients require effective treatment. People with malnutrition need to adjust to a balanced diet, and so on. The speed of weight loss is a key factor in determining the improvement or deterioration of liver histology.

9.1 Lifestyle

Because the etiology and pathogenesis of NAFLD are unknown, there is no effective drug therapy for liver disease. None of NASH drugs are currently in Phase III clinical trials, and there are no drugs approved by government regulators to treat NASH.

For obese patients with fatty liver, diet therapy is the basis and key approach. Lifestyle modification is recommended as the primary treatment for NAFLD [60]. For NAFLD patients who are overweight or obese (abdominal obesity), the first optional lifestyle is aimed at weight loss with a range of 8–10%. More than 50% of patients fail to meet the target and require individualized drug treatment. NAFLD patients should adjust their diet, which should be supplemented with high protein, an appropriate amount of fat, and sugar with rationally allocated. The total energy intake should be controlled at about 20–25 kcal per kilogram per day. Meanwhile, patients should strictly control their daily salt intake, avoid foods rich in monosaccharides and disaccharides, such as high-sugar pastries, ice cream, candies, etc.

Exercise is very important in the treatment of NAFLD. It is recommended that patients should take aerobic exercise, such as jogging, brisk walking, swimming, and so on. The specific time and amount of each and gradual exercise need to be personalized. Weight loss is generally controlled at 0.5–1 kg/week because losing weight too quickly is also harmful to the body.

9.2 Obesity management

Weight loss should be a priority in obese patients and those with MetS. Obesity can be addressed through lifestyle changes such as a low-calorie diet with an adequate intake of fruits and vegetables and increased physical activity. Although medical treatment and bariatric surgery may also be considered, however, the adverse effects cannot be eliminated.

9.3 Pharmacotherapy for patients with T2DM

NAFLD is an acquired metabolic stress-induced liver injury closely associated with IR and genetic susceptibility. The metabolic disorders in T2DM patients are similar to NAFLD. Therefore, the glucose metabolism in T2DM patients with NAFLD will further deteriorate, making diabetes difficult to control, and requiring more hypoglycemic drug treatment. Metformin is the preferred treatment for patients with T2DM unless there is a specific contraindication, such as in patients with renal impairment.

Since metformin does not promote insulin secretion, it generally does not cause hypoglycemia when used alone. Animal and in vitro studies have shown that metformin has a protective effect against several T2DM-related cardiovascular diseases, including myocardial infarction, hypertrophic, and diabetic cardiomyopathy, which lead to cardiac insufficiency and the potential progression to heart failure. The molecular mechanisms involved in this protection are multifaceted and function primarily by acting on vascular endothelial cells, cardiomyocytes, and fibroblasts. Since metformin is excreted by the kidney, the accumulation of metformin and lactic acid easily occurs in the body when the kidney functions insufficiently, increasing the risk of acidosis thereby. The doctors generally recommend cessation when the serum creatinine is greater than 150 micromol/liter. In addition, the drug should also be discontinued when there is severe cardiac and liver dysfunction, and the liver and kidney functions should be checked regularly during the medication.

Sulfonylureas, such as gliclazide and glimepiride, act on β cells to stimulate insulin secretion and increase the level of insulin in the body. Some sulfonylurea drugs (such as glimepiride) can enhance the sensitivity of peripheral tissues to insulin, reduce the output of hepatic glycogen, and also have the effect of reducing platelet aggregation, regulating blood lipids and blood viscosity, and improving blood circulation (e.g., gliclazide). Sulfonylureas boost the production of insulin, a hormone that promotes energy storage, which may indirectly contribute to weight gain. Among various sulfonylureas, clinical studies have shown that glipizide controlled-release tablets and glimepiride have no significant effect on weight gain. Metformin, acarbose, and sodium-glucose cotransporter 2 (SGLT-2) inhibitors also have weight loss effects. For overweight or obese patients, sulfonylureas in combination with these drugs may reduce the risk of weight gain associated with sulfonylureas.

NAFLD patients with diabetes should have effective improvement not only in NASH, but also in NAFLD-related MetS, T2DM, and cardiovascular diseases. In the treatment of NASH, it is necessary to take effective measures to lose 8–10% of body weight, including lifestyle intervention. If the standard is not met, drug treatment can be selected. Patients eligible for bariatric surgery may also be considered.

9.4 Gut flora

In addition to genetic susceptibility and diet, the gut microbiota influences hepatic carbohydrate, lipid metabolism, and the balance between pro-and anti-inflammatory cytokines in the liver, thereby affecting NAFLD and its progression to NASH. Hyperproliferation of intestinal bacteria can lead to changes in cytokines in the portal vein and liver, so probiotics and antibiotics may help treat this disease. Animal experiments have shown that probiotics can down-regulate TNF-α levels and reduce liver inflammation, but clinical studies are needed to confirm the efficacy. Antibiotics that are not absorbed in the gut may be helpful in the treatment of intestinal bacterial hyperproliferation. Rifaximin, which is rarely absorbed in the gut, is well tolerated and may have certain advantages [61]. However, there is no randomized controlled clinical study to observe the efficacy of antibiotics on NAFLD.

9.5 Potential drugs

Studies have found that liver fibrosis can be reversed in a series of processes including the occurrence and development of NAFLD. The activation of HSCs to produce collagen is the core link of liver fibrosis. Although great progress has been made in the study of HSCs activation-related genes, few breakthroughs are achieved in the treatment of liver fibrosis, and the search for effective anti-fibrosis drugs is still a research hotspot. By choosing appropriate drugs, the clinical prognosis of NAFLD can be optimal, which has important social and economic significance.

9.5.1 Curcumin

Turmeric is the dried rhizome of turmeric (*Curcuma longa* L.), which has been used in traditional medicine in China for thousands of years and is widely used in flavoring, dyeing, and pharmaceutical industries. The main active ingredient is a class of diarylheptane compounds derived from ginger plants, which mainly exist in the rhizomes of medicinal plants such as turmeric, tulip, and Curcuma. At present, more than 40 kinds of Curcumin compounds have been isolated from the genus Curcuma, among which Curcumin is the main active substance, and the main chain is unsaturated aliphatic and aromatic groups. Since it was first isolated from plants in 1870 but its molecular structure was determined in 1910, years of research have found that it has a variety of biological functions, such as regulating blood lipids, anti-tumor, anti-virus, and anti-inflammatory effects, and act as antioxidants. Through research on the mechanism and intervention of NAFLD-related hepatic stellate cell activation, it is of great theoretical significance to clarify the potential mechanism of Curcumin to inhibit the occurrence of hepatic fibrosis.

Liver fibrosis is a wound repair response to chronic liver injury (viral infection, alcoholism, cholestasis, etc.), and is a pathological process of excessive extracellular matrix (ECM) production and deposition. Chronic liver injury leads to the accumulation of a large number of inflammatory cells, which release inflammatory factors and growth factors, such as TNF-α and TGF-β1, thereby activating HSCs, which are generated by ECM (especially collagen fibers). Curcumin has received great attention as a dietary supplement for liver protection. Curcumin can inhibit the activities of lipoxygenase and cyclooxygenase-2 (COX-2), inhibit lipid peroxidation, reduce the release of arachidonic acid, especially the inflammatory factors ILs by inhibiting the NF-kB signaling pathway—production of 1β, IL-6, TNF-α. Our previous findings provide new insights into the mechanism of action of curcumin and a therapeutic candidate for the prevention and treatment of hyperleptinemia-induced liver fibrosis in NASH patients with obesity and/or T2DM [62–64]. In recent years, several in vitro and in vivo studies have also shown that curcumin can intervene in the pathological process of liver diseases from multiple links, and has anti-hepatic injury, anti-steatosis, anti-fibrosis, and anti-cancer effects. However, due to the poor water solubility and low bioavailability of curcumin, its clinical application is greatly limited. Therefore, the formulation and structural modification of curcumin as a lead compound are currently hot and crucial research topics.

9.5.2 Vitamin E

Vitamin E is a fat-soluble vitamin with antioxidant function, which is necessary for the normal growth and reproduction of animals. Studies have found that vitamin

E has a similar biological activity to a-tocopherol, which can provide a hydrogen ion on the color ring to scavenge free radicals, thereby playing an anti-oxidative stress role. In addition to scavenging reactive oxygen free radicals, vitamin E can also scavenge reactive nitrogen free radicals. Both of them play important roles in the occurrence and development of NAFLD. In vivo experiments in mice found that vitamin E plays an important regulatory role in improving glucose and lipid metabolism, and vitamin E supplementation can significantly improve lipid metabolism in NAFLD mice. Clinical trials have found that vitamin E supplementation can significantly improve liver pathological outcomes in non-diabetic NAFLD patients [65]. However, there was no significant improvement in diabetic patients with NAFLD [66]. Therefore, vitamin E therapy can be considered for non-diabetic NASH patients who have failed lifestyle interventions.

9.5.3 Peroxisome proliferator-activated receptor alpha (PPAR-α) agonist

Peroxisome proliferator-activated receptors (PPARs) are members of the nuclear receptor superfamily of ligand-activated transcription factors. PPARs contain three isoforms consisting of PPARα, PPARβ/δ, and PPARγ. Among them, PPARα is abundantly expressed in hepatocytes. PPARα has a key role in regulating fatty acid transport as well as peroxisomal and mitochondrial β-oxidation in the liver. The researchers found that PPARα expression in the human liver was inversely correlated with the severity of NAFLD. Currently, PPARα-agonists have been shown to improve IR and significantly increase energy expenditure. PPARα-agonists improve pathological conditions in a NAFLD mouse model by modulating lipid turnover and energy metabolism in the liver [67].

9.5.4 Farnesoid X receptor agonists

Farnesoid X Receptor (FXR) is a bile acid receptor, a member of the nuclear receptor superfamily. Studies have found that the nuclear receptor transcription factor FXR can participate in the regulation of various metabolic pathways through the regulation of its corresponding target genes. FXR and retinol X receptor (RXR) bind to the FXR response element in the promoter region of target genes in the form of heterodimers to regulate the transcription of downstream genes. Fibroblast growth factor 21 (FGF21) is an important cytokine downstream of FXR that regulates glucose and lipid metabolism in the body. It can enhance the hydrolysis of adipose tissue, thereby increasing the rate of fatty acid oxidation. Activation of FXR by bile acids can increase the expression and secretion of FGF21, and the increased expression of FGF21 can reduce the content of triglycerides in the liver. Therefore, it can be used as an important drug target for NAFLD [68]. Obeticholic acid is a kind of FXR. In a phase 3 study in the treatment of NAFLD, 25 mg of Obeticholic acid significantly improved fibrosis in NASH patients [69]. Therefore, FXR agonists may also be considered as one of the potential drugs for NAFLD.

10. Future prospects

Several issues related to NAFLD require further research to clarify. Furthermore, the lack of understanding of the pathogenesis, causality, and genetic factors of NAFLD have hindered the development of new therapeutics. Therefore, further basic and clinical studies are needed to better understand the development of NAFLD from the perspectives of genetic, molecular, and cell signaling, etc. Focusing on the underlying mechanisms may be valuable in identifying new therapeutic targets for metabolic diseases. Lifestyle interventions are the recommended initial therapy for the treatment of NAFLD. To date, there is insufficient evidence to support the use of drugs that primarily target the underlying causes of MetS. Therefore, if lifestyle changes are not sufficient, other measures that target individual risk factors may be needed. Most importantly, improved strategies are needed to achieve and maintain long-term weight loss and increased physical activity. In future research, not only basic medical research will be conducted but also actively innovate and carry out translational medicines. It is believed that with the joint efforts of medicinal chemists and clinical experts, new drugs will be used in the treatment of liver diseases.

Acknowledgements

This work is supported by research grants from the National Natural Science Foundation of China (31471330), National Key R&D Program of China (2020YFC2006100 and 2020YFC2006101), National Key R&D Program of China (2020YFC2009000 and 2020YFC2009006), Henan Provincial Key R&D and Promotion Special Project (212102310033), Zhengzhou University Discipline Key Special Project (XKZDQY202001). Furthermore, we thank Dr. Ihtisham Bukhari (Gastroenterology, The Fifth Affiliated Hospital, Zhengzhou University, Zhengzhou, Henan, China) for his linguistic assistance.

Conflict of interest

The authors declare no conflict of interest.

Author details

Youcai Tang[1,2,3,4,5*], Xuecui Yin[2] and Yuying Ma[2]

1 Department of Pediatrics, The Fifth Affiliated Hospital, Zhengzhou University, Zhengzhou, Henan, China

2 Gastroenterology, The Fifth Affiliated Hospital, Zhengzhou University, Zhengzhou, Henan, China

3 Henan Key Laboratory of Rehabilitation Medicine, The Fifth Affiliated Hospital, Zhengzhou University, Zhengzhou, Henan, China

4 Henan Joint International Research Laboratory of Chronic Liver Injury, The Fifth Affiliated Hospital, Zhengzhou University, Zhengzhou, Henan, China

5 Zhengzhou Key Laboratory of Metabolic-dysfunction-associated Fatty Liver Disease, The Fifth Affiliated Hospital, Zhengzhou University, Zhengzhou, Henan, China

*Address all correspondence to: tangyoucai@hotmail.com

References

[1] Eslam M, Newsome PN, Sarin SK, et al. A new definition for metabolic dysfunction-associated fatty liver disease: An international expert consensus statement. Journal of Hepatology. 2020;**73**(1):202-209. DOI: 10.1016/j.jhep.2020.03.039

[2] Younossi Z, Tacke F, Arrese M, et al. Global perspectives on nonalcoholic fatty liver disease and nonalcoholic steatohepatitis. Hepatology. 2019;**69**(6): 2672-2682. DOI: 10.1002/hep.30251

[3] Zhou F, Zhou J, Wang W, et al. Unexpected rapid increase in the burden of NAFLD in China from 2008 to 2018: A systematic review and meta-analysis. Hepatology. 2019;**70**(4):1119-1133. DOI: 10.1002/hep.30702

[4] Shetty D, Amarapurkar A, Shukla A. Primary versus secondary NAFLD: Perspective on advanced fibrosis. Journal of Clinical and Experimental Hepatology. 2021;**11**(5):557-564. DOI: 10.1016/j.jceh.2020.12.009

[5] Blüher M. Metabolically healthy obesity. Endocrine Reviews. 2020;**41**: 3. DOI: 10.1210/endrev/bnaa004

[6] Lee JJ, Pedley A, Hoffmann U, Massaro JM, Levy D, Long MT. Visceral and intrahepatic fat are associated with cardiometabolic risk factors above other ectopic fat depots: The Framingham heart study. The American Journal of Medicine. 2018;**131**(6):684-692.e612. DOI: 10.1016/j.amjmed.2018.02.002

[7] Du K, Murakami S, Sun Y, Kilpatrick CL, Luscher B. DHHC7 palmitoylates glucose transporter 4 (Glut4) and regulates Glut4 membrane translocation. The Journal of Biological Chemistry. 2017;**292**(7):2979-2991. DOI: 10.1074/jbc.M116.747139

[8] Musovic S, Olofsson CS. Adrenergic stimulation of adiponectin secretion in visceral mouse adipocytes is blunted in high-fat diet induced obesity. Scientific Reports. 2019;**9**(1):10680. DOI: 10.1038/s41598-019-47113-8

[9] Cohen P, Kajimura S. The cellular and functional complexity of thermogenic fat. Nature Reviews. Molecular Cell Biology. 2021;**22**(6):393-409. DOI: 10.1038/s41580-021-00350-0

[10] Rosso C, Kazankov K, Younes R, et al. Crosstalk between adipose tissue insulin resistance and liver macrophages in non-alcoholic fatty liver disease. Journal of Hepatology. 2019;**71**(5):1012-1021. DOI: 10.1016/j.jhep.2019.06.031

[11] Beals JW, Smith GI, Shankaran M, et al. Increased adipose tissue fibrogenesis, not impaired expandability, is associated with nonalcoholic fatty liver disease. Hepatology. 2021;**74**(3): 1287-1299. DOI: 10.1002/hep.31822

[12] Petersen MC, Shulman GI. Mechanisms of insulin action and insulin resistance. Physiological Reviews. 2018;**98**(4):2133-2223. DOI: 10.1152/physrev.00063.2017

[13] Rorsman P, Ashcroft FM. Pancreatic β-cell electrical activity and insulin secretion: Of mice and men. Physiological Reviews. 2018;**98**(1):117-214. DOI: 10.1152/physrev.00008.2017

[14] Tuttle KR, Brosius FC 3rd, Cavender MA, et al. SGLT2 inhibition for CKD and cardiovascular disease in type 2 diabetes: Report of a scientific workshop sponsored by the National Kidney Foundation. Diabetes. 2021;**70**(1):1-16. DOI: 10.2337/dbi20-0040

[15] Rhee JJ, Jardine MJ, Chertow GM, Mahaffey KW. Dedicated kidney disease-focused outcome trials with sodium-glucose cotransporter-2 inhibitors: Lessons from CREDENCE and expectations from DAPA-HF, DAPA-CKD, and EMPA-KIDNEY. Diabetes, Obesity & Metabolism. 2020;**22**(Suppl. 1): 46-54. DOI: 10.1111/dom.13987

[16] Murai J, Nishizawa H, Otsuka A, et al. Low muscle quality in Japanese type 2 diabetic patients with visceral fat accumulation. Cardiovascular Diabetology. 2018;**17**(1):112. DOI: 10.1186/s12933-018-0755-3

[17] Leite NC, Villela-Nogueira CA, Pannain VL, et al. Histopathological stages of nonalcoholic fatty liver disease in type 2 diabetes: Prevalences and correlated factors. Liver International. 2011;**31**(5):700-706. DOI: 10.1111/j.1478-3231.2011.02482.x

[18] Farrell G, Schattenberg JM, Leclercq I, et al. Mouse models of nonalcoholic steatohepatitis: Toward optimization of their relevance to human nonalcoholic steatohepatitis. Hepatology. 2019;**69**(5):2241-2257. DOI: 10.1002/hep.30333

[19] Tune JD, Goodwill AG, Sassoon DJ, Mather KJ. Cardiovascular consequences of metabolic syndrome. Translational Research. 2017;**183**:57-70. DOI: 10.1016/j.trsl.2017.01.001

[20] Alberti KG, Eckel RH, Grundy SM, et al. Harmonizing the metabolic syndrome: A joint interim statement of the international diabetes federation task force on epidemiology and prevention; National Heart, Lung, and Blood Institute; American Heart Association; World Heart Federation; International Atherosclerosis Society; and International Association for the Study of Obesity. Circulation. 2009;**120**(16):1640-1645. DOI: 10.1161/circulationaha.109.192644

[21] Friedman SL, Neuschwander-Tetri BA, Rinella M, Sanyal AJ. Mechanisms of NAFLD development and therapeutic strategies. Nature Medicine. 2018;**24**(7):908-922. DOI: 10.1038/s41591-018-0104-9

[22] Fan JG, Kim SU, Wong VW. New trends on obesity and NAFLD in Asia. Journal of Hepatology. 2017;**67**(4): 862-873. DOI: 10.1016/j.jhep.2017.06.003

[23] Eslam M, Valenti L, Romeo S. Genetics and epigenetics of NAFLD and NASH: Clinical impact. Journal of Hepatology. 2018;**68**(2):268-279. DOI: 10.1016/j.jhep.2017.09.003

[24] Wang Q, Ou X, Jia J, et al. Association between polymorphism of PNPLA3 rs738409 and severity of fibrosis in adult nonalcoholic fatty liver disease. Journal of Clinical and Experimental Medicine. 2020;**19**(14):1464-1467. DOI: 10.1097/MD.0000000000014324

[25] Cai W, Weng D, Ling S, Wang S, Ma L, Yao H. Association between nonalcoholic fatty liver disease and interaction of PNPLA3-rs738409 polymorphism and smoking in Uyghur population. Practical Preventive Medicine. 2018;**25**(05):517-519, 575. DOI: 10.3969/j.issn.1006-3110.2018.05.002

[26] Kozlitina J, Smagris E, Stender S, et al. Exome-wide association study identifies a TM6SF2 variant that confers susceptibility to nonalcoholic fatty liver disease. Nature Genetics. 2014;**46**(4):352-356. DOI: 10.1038/ng.2901

[27] Tripathi A, Debelius J, Brenner DA, et al. The gut-liver axis and the intersection with the microbiome.

Nature Reviews. Gastroenterology & Hepatology. 2018;**15**(7):397-411. DOI: 10.1038/s41575-018-0011-z

[28] Marra F, Svegliati-Baroni G. Lipotoxicity and the gut-liver axis in NASH pathogenesis. Journal of Hepatology. 2018;**68**(2):280-295. DOI: 10.1016/j.jhep.2017.11.014

[29] Ma KL, Ruan XZ, Powis SH, Chen Y, Moorhead JF, Varghese Z. Inflammatory stress exacerbates lipid accumulation in hepatic cells and fatty livers of apolipoprotein E knockout mice. Hepatology. 2008;**48**(3):770-781. DOI: 10.1002/hep.22423

[30] Buzzetti E, Pinzani M, Tsochatzis EA. The multiple-hit pathogenesis of non-alcoholic fatty liver disease (NAFLD). Metabolism. 2016;**65**(8):1038-1048. DOI: 10.1016/j.metabol.2015.12.012

[31] Haeusler RA, McGraw TE, Accili D. Biochemical and cellular properties of insulin receptor signalling. Nature Reviews. Molecular Cell Biology. 2018;**19**(1):31-44. DOI: 10.1038/nrm.2017.89

[32] Haythorne E, Rohm M, van de Bunt M, et al. Diabetes causes marked inhibition of mitochondrial metabolism in pancreatic β-cells. Nature Communications. 2019;**10**(1):2474. DOI: 10.1038/s41467-019-10189-x

[33] Brunt EM, Wong VW, Nobili V, et al. Nonalcoholic fatty liver disease. Nature Reviews. Disease Primers. 2015;**1**:15080. DOI: 10.1038/nrdp.2015.80

[34] Stumvoll M, Goldstein BJ, van Haeften TW. Type 2 diabetes: Principles of pathogenesis and therapy. Lancet. 2005;**365**(9467):1333-1346. DOI: 10.1016/s0140-6736(05)61032-x

[35] Wang M, Kaufman RJ. Protein misfolding in the endoplasmic reticulum as a conduit to human disease. Nature. 2016;**529**(7586):326-335. DOI: 10.1038/nature17041

[36] Walter P, Ron D. The unfolded protein response: From stress pathway to homeostatic regulation. Science. 2011;**334**(6059):1081-1086. DOI: 10.1126/science.1209038

[37] Urano F, Wang X, Bertolotti A, et al. Coupling of stress in the ER to activation of JNK protein kinases by transmembrane protein kinase IRE1. Science. 2000;**287**(5453):664-666. DOI: 10.1126/science.287.5453.664

[38] Malhi H, Kaufman RJ. Endoplasmic reticulum stress in liver disease. Journal of Hepatology. 2011;**54**(4):795-809. DOI: 10.1016/j.jhep.2010.11.005

[39] Nath B, Levin I, Csak T, et al. Hepatocyte-specific hypoxia-inducible factor-1α is a determinant of lipid accumulation and liver injury in alcohol-induced steatosis in mice. Hepatology. 2011;**53**(5):1526-1537. DOI: 10.1002/hep.24256

[40] Cobbina E, Akhlaghi F. Non-alcoholic fatty liver disease (NAFLD) - pathogenesis, classification, and effect on drug metabolizing enzymes and transporters. Drug Metabolism Reviews. 2017;**49**(2):197-211. DOI: 10.1080/03602532.2017.1293683

[41] Zimmermann E, Anty R, Tordjman J, et al. C-reactive protein levels in relation to various features of non-alcoholic fatty liver disease among obese patients. Journal of Hepatology. 2011;**55**(3):660-665. DOI: 10.1016/j.jhep.2010.12.017

[42] Singh P, Peterson TE, Sert-Kuniyoshi FH, et al. Leptin signaling in adipose tissue: Role in lipid accumulation

and weight gain. Circulation Research. 2012;**111**(5):599-603. DOI: 10.1161/circresaha.112.273656

[43] Tang Y. Curcumin targets multiple pathways to halt hepatic stellate cell activation: Updated mechanisms in vitro and in vivo. Digestive Diseases and Sciences. 2015;**60**(6):1554-1564. DOI: 10.1007/s10620-014-3487-6

[44] Leshan RL, Greenwald-Yarnell M, Patterson CM, Gonzalez IE, Myers MG Jr. Leptin action through hypothalamic nitric oxide synthase-1-expressing neurons controls energy balance. Nature Medicine. 2012;**18**(5):820-823. DOI: 10.1038/nm.2724

[45] Kwon O, Kim KW, Kim MS. Leptin signalling pathways in hypothalamic neurons. Cellular and Molecular Life Sciences. 2016;**73**(7):1457-1477. DOI: 10.1007/s00018-016-2133-1

[46] Fang H, Judd RL. Adiponectin regulation and function. Comprehensive Physiology. 2018;**8**(3):1031-1063. DOI: 10.1002/cphy.c170046

[47] Okada-Iwabu M, Yamauchi T, Iwabu M, et al. A small-molecule AdipoR agonist for type 2 diabetes and short life in obesity. Nature. 2013;**503**(7477):493-499. DOI: 10.1038/nature12656

[48] Adachi M, Brenner DA. High molecular weight adiponectin inhibits proliferation of hepatic stellate cells via activation of adenosine monophosphate-activated protein kinase. Hepatology. 2008;**47**(2):677-685. DOI: 10.1002/hep.21991

[49] Puche JE, Saiman Y, Friedman SL. Hepatic stellate cells and liver fibrosis. Comprehensive Physiology. 2013;**3**(4):1473-1492. DOI: 10.1002/cphy.c120035

[50] Wang Y, Gao J, Zhang D, Zhang J, Ma J, Jiang H. New insights into the antifibrotic effects of sorafenib on hepatic stellate cells and liver fibrosis. Journal of Hepatology. 2010;**53**(1):132-144. DOI: 10.1016/j.jhep.2010.02.027

[51] Gao J, Wei B, de Assuncao TM, et al. Hepatic stellate cell autophagy inhibits extracellular vesicle release to attenuate liver fibrosis. Journal of Hepatology. 2020;**73**(5):1144-1154. DOI: 10.1016/j.jhep.2020.04.044

[52] Singal AK, Bataller R, Ahn J, Kamath PS, Shah VH. ACG clinical guideline: Alcoholic liver disease. The American Journal of Gastroenterology. 2018;**113**(2):175-194. DOI: 10.1038/ajg.2017.469

[53] Bajaj JS. Alcohol, liver disease and the gut microbiota. Nature Reviews. Gastroenterology & Hepatology. 2019;**16**(4):235-246. DOI: 10.1038/s41575-018-0099-1

[54] Sarin SK, Kumar M, Eslam M, et al. Liver diseases in the Asia-Pacific region: A Lancet Gastroenterology & Hepatology Commission. The Lancet Gastroenterology & Hepatology. 2020;**5**(2):167-228. DOI: 10.1016/s2468-1253(19)30342-5

[55] EASL. 2017 clinical practice guidelines on the management of hepatitis B virus infection. Journal of Hepatology. 2017;**67**(2):370-398. DOI: 10.1016/j.jhep.2017.03.021

[56] Chen DY, Wolski D, Aneja J, et al. Hepatitis C virus-specific CD4+ T cell phenotype and function in different infection outcomes. The Journal of Clinical Investigation. 2020;**130**(2):768-773. DOI: 10.1172/jci126277

[57] Mieli-Vergani G, Vergani D, Czaja AJ, et al. Autoimmune hepatitis. Nature

Reviews Disease Primers. 2018;**4**:18017. DOI: 10.1038/nrdp.2018.17

[58] Galaski J, Weiler-Normann C, Schakat M, et al. Update of the simplified criteria for autoimmune hepatitis: Evaluation of the methodology for immunoserological testing. Journal of Hepatology. 2021;**74**(2):312-320. DOI: 10.1016/j.jhep.2020.07.032

[59] Członkowska A, Litwin T, Dusek P, et al. Wilson disease. Nature Reviews Disease Primers. 2018;**4**(1):21. DOI: 10.1038/s41572-018-0018-3

[60] Sheka AC, Adeyi O, Thompson J, Hameed B, Crawford PA, Ikramuddin S. Nonalcoholic steatohepatitis: A review. Journal of the American Medical Association. 2020;**323**(12):1175-1183. DOI: 10.1001/jama.2020.2298

[61] Cobbold JFL, Atkinson S, Marchesi JR, et al. Rifaximin in non-alcoholic steatohepatitis: An open-label pilot study. Hepatology Research. 2018;**48**(1):69-77. DOI: 10.1111/hepr.12904

[62] Tang Y, Chen A. Curcumin eliminates the effect of advanced glycation end-products (AGEs) on the divergent regulation of gene expression of receptors of AGEs by interrupting leptin signaling. Laboratory Investigation. 2014;**94**(5):503-516. DOI: 10.1038/labinvest.2014.42

[63] Lin J, Tang Y, Kang Q, Chen A. Curcumin eliminates the inhibitory effect of advanced glycation end-products (AGEs) on gene expression of AGE receptor-1 in hepatic stellate cells in vitro. Laboratory Investigation. 2012;**92**(6):827-841. DOI: 10.1038/labinvest.2012.53

[64] Tang Y, Chen A. Curcumin prevents leptin raising glucose levels in hepatic stellate cells by blocking translocation of glucose transporter-4 and increasing glucokinase. British Journal of Pharmacology. 2010;**161**(5):1137-1149. DOI: 10.1111/j.1476-5381.2010.00956.x

[65] Violi F, Cangemi R. Pioglitazone, vitamin E, or placebo for nonalcoholic steatohepatitis. The New England Journal of Medicine. 2010;**363**(12):1185-1186; author reply 1186. DOI: 10.1056/NEJMc1006581

[66] Bril F, Biernacki DM, Kalavalapalli S, et al. Role of vitamin E for nonalcoholic steatohepatitis in patients with type 2 diabetes: A randomized controlled trial. Diabetes Care. 2019;**42**(8):1481-1488. DOI: 10.2337/dc19-0167

[67] Honda Y, Kessoku T, Ogawa Y, et al. Pemafibrate, a novel selective peroxisome proliferator-activated receptor alpha modulator, improves the pathogenesis in a rodent model of nonalcoholic steatohepatitis. Scientific Reports. 2017;7:42477. DOI: 10.1038/srep42477

[68] Sumida Y, Yoneda M. Current and future pharmacological therapies for NAFLD/NASH. Journal of Gastroenterology. 2018;**53**(3):362-376. DOI: 10.1007/s00535-017-1415-1

[69] Younossi ZM, Ratziu V, Loomba R, et al. Obeticholic acid for the treatment of non-alcoholic steatohepatitis: Interim analysis from a multicentre, randomised, placebo-controlled phase 3 trial. Lancet. 2019;**394**(10215):2184-2196. DOI: 10.1016/s0140-6736(19)33041-7

Chapter 7

Hepatocellular Carcinoma

Rahmat Adetutu Adisa and Lateef Adegboyega Sulaimon

Abstract

Over 1 million cases of liver cancer are estimated to occur by 2025, making it a global health challenge. In almost 90% of cases of liver cancer, it is hepatocellular carcinoma (HCC). The main risk factors for HCC development are infection with hepatitis B and C viruses, although nonalcoholic steatohepatitis (NASH) associated with metabolic syndrome or diabetes mellitus is becoming more prevalent in the West. The molecular pathogenesis of nonalcoholic steatohepatitis-associated HCC is unique. A quarter of all HCCs present with mutations that are potentially actionable but have not yet been translated into clinical practice. In the advanced stages of the disease, systemic therapy is expected to be administered 50–60% of the time to HCC patients. In phase III trials, six systemic therapies have been approved (atezolizumab plus bevacizumab, sorafenib, lenvatinib, regorafenib, cabozantinib, and ramucirumab), and new trials are evaluating combination therapies, such as checkpoint inhibitors and tyrosine kinase inhibitors or anti-VEGF therapies. The findings of these clinical trials are expected to alter the landscape of managing HCC at all stages of the disease.

Keywords: hepatocellular carcinoma, nonalcoholic steatohepatitis, hepatitis B, hepatitis C, systemic therapies

1. Introduction

The incidence of liver cancer is growing worldwide [1, 2] and research estimates that millions of people will be affected by the disease annually by 2025 [3]. Hepatocellular carcinoma (HCC) describes the most common type of liver cancer, responsible for nearly 90% of all cases. The most significant risk factor for HCC development is infection with the hepatitis B virus (HBV), accounting for 50% of all cases [4]. With antiviral drugs, patients have achieved sustained virological response (SVR), reducing the risk of hepatitis C virus (HCV) infection substantially [5]. Nevertheless, the risk of HCC for individuals with cirrhosis remains even after HCV clearance. Nonalcoholic steatohepatitis (NASH) is becoming the main cause of HCC in the West, since it is associated with metabolic syndrome and diabetes mellitus [6]. Furthermore, there have also been reports that aristolochic acid and tobacco are potentially pathogenic cofactors for HCC [7].

The incidence of HCC differs depending on the etiology and type of genotoxins, although there is a greater understanding of the pathophysiology and drivers of HCC over the past few years; clinical applications of these insights have yet to emerge. There are actionable mutations of HCC tumors in approximately 25% of cases;

however, most mutations are less than 10%, making proof-of-concept studies difficult [7, 8]. The majority of mutations in HCC remain unsolvable, including those in TERT, TP53, and CTNNB1 [9]. Researchers are also still working on how to establish biomarkers that guide therapy based on molecular and immune classes.

Since the early 2010s, HCC management has vastly improved [8, 10–12]. The mainstay curative treatments in HCC cases have been hepatic resection and liver transplantation. For tumors down-staged beyond Milan criteria, refinements in patient selection have led to improved surgical resection results and outstanding 10-year post-liver transplantation survival rates [10, 13]. In nonsurgical early-stage HCCs, image-guided ablation using radiofrequency remains the gold standard despite advancements in alternative approaches [12]. Following these potentially curative methods, adjuvant therapies to prevent relapse are an unmet medical need, as randomized controlled trials (RCTs) have so far given poor results. The most frequently used and standard treatment for intermediate-stage HCC for the past two decades has been transarterial chemoembolization (TACE) [14]. Transarterial radioembolization (TARE) has been demonstrated to be effective in phase II studies [15], but guidelines have not yet established it as a primary standard of therapy. The arsenal of intermediate therapy is unlikely to improve in the immediate term with more locoregional devices or radiation oncology methods.

There has been a threat to the use of traditional HCC treatments from systemic medicines, such as tyrosine kinase inhibitors (TKIs), immune checkpoint inhibitors (ICIs), and monoclonal antibodies. Patients with HCC are predicted to be exposed to systemic therapy 50–60% of the time over their lives, especially in advanced stages of the disease [8]. The development of systemic medicines has progressed dramatically in the last 5 years, with studies showing significant improvements in overall survival and quality of life for patients [8]. As a result of the combination of anti-PDL1 antibody atezolizumab and anti-VEGF antibody bevacizumab, patients with advanced-stage HCC have a quadrupled life expectancy and improved patient-reported outcomes [16]. The most successful single-drug therapies are still sorafenib [17] and lenvatinib [18]. Regorafenib [19], cabozantinib [20], and ramucirumab [21] have similarly shown enhanced survival advantages when switched to single-agent regimens. In 15–20% of responders, single-agent ICIs produce significant therapeutic advantages, although biomarkers have thus far failed to identify this group [22, 23]. Phase III trials are also underway that examine combinations of ICIs with TKIs or PD1/PDL1 axis inhibitors with CTLA4 inhibitors to examine the efficacy of these therapies. The findings of these studies are expected to alter the landscape of managing HCC at all stages of the disease.

2. Epidemiology of HCC

In 2018, there were 841,080 new cases of liver cancer, making it the sixth most common cancer worldwide and the fourth leading cause of cancer-related death [3]. Despite an increase in HCC incidence and mortality in different parts of Europe and the United States [24], the highest rates are seen in East Asia and Africa. SEER reports that HCC has been the fastest-growing cancer-related cause of death in the United States since the early 2000s. HCC is expected to be the third leading cause of cancer-related death by 2030 if current trends continue [25].

3. Risk factors of HCC

Chronic liver disease is responsible for more than 90% of all cases of HCC. All forms of cirrhosis are major risk factors for HCC [10, 11]. Annually, 1–6% of patients with cirrhosis die of HCC. HBV and HCV infection, chronic alcohol consumption, and diabetes- or obesity-related NASH all increase the risk for HCC [26]. Hemochromatosis, antitrypsin deficiency, and cirrhosis from primary biliary cholangitis all represent less common risk factors for HCC. Up to 45% of people with hemochromatosis who develop cirrhosis over their lifetime will develop HCC [27].

4. Hepatitis B viral infection

The cause of HCC in Asia and Africa is 60% HBV infection, while it is 20% in the West [4]. HBV is a DNA virus that can cause insertional mutagenesis and activate oncogenes by integrating into the host genome [28]. HBV increases the risk of liver cancer even if there is no cirrhosis in most patients with HBV-induced HCC. Due to the high prevalence of endemic HBV in East Asia, males (40 years of age) and females (50 years of age) have a high risk of developing HCC, which necessitates surveillance programs. The incidence of HCC in patients in their early 30s or 40s in Africa is likely due to their exposure to aflatoxin B1, a carcinogen, which increases the risk of developing HCC in combination with HBV [29]. Many Asian countries still do not have universal immunization programs, despite the fact that HBV vaccination programs have reduced HCC incidence in some regions [30].

5. Hepatitis C viral infection

The most common underlying liver disease in North America, Europe, and Japan is chronic HCV infection [4]. In contrast to HBV, HCV is an RNA virus that does not integrate into the host genome, so those who develop cirrhosis or chronic liver disease with bridging fibrosis are at risk of developing HCC. Direct-acting antiviral (DAA) medications have enabled more and more people to achieve a sustained viral response (SVR), thereby reducing their risk of developing HCC by 50–80% [5]. A number of patients, especially those from minority racial or ethnic groups and those from low-income socioeconomic areas, have not been tested for HCV and thus have no idea of their infection [31]. Additionally, people with HCV-induced cirrhosis remain at risk of developing HCC even after they have achieved sustained virologic response (>2% per year) and, thus, they have to be monitored closely [32, 33].

6. Hepatitis D viral infection

HBV surface antigens are necessary for HDV to replicate and infect. HDV is an RNA virus. Twenty to forty million people are estimated to be infected with HDV worldwide, and these individuals experience more severe liver disease, notably fibrosis and cirrhosis, than people who have only HBV. Furthermore, several cohort studies have found that co-infection with HDV and HBV may lead to an increased risk of HCC than HBV infection alone. A study reported that patients with acute or chronic HDV infection were at a significantly higher risk of HCC than those with a sole HBV infection [34].

7. Alcohol

A fatty liver, cirrhosis, and HCC are all caused by excessive alcohol consumption. Cirrhosis caused by persistent alcohol consumption, also known as NASH, is becoming increasingly common. HCC is associated with alcohol-induced cirrhosis in 15–30% of cases depending on geographic region, with an annual incidence varying between 1% observed in population-based studies and 2–3% recorded in tertiary care referral centers [35]. There is also evidence that chronic alcohol consumption increases the risk of HCC from other causes; for example, several studies suggest that those who drink alcohol and are HBV carriers are more likely to develop HCC [36]. Although alcohol consumption has some similarities with other forms of cirrhosis, particularly NASH, in some pathophysiological processes, there is an indication that alcohol consumption may have different pro-tumorigenic mechanisms in individuals.

8. Nonalcoholic steatohepatitis (NASH)

Patients with diabetes mellitus or obesity may also develop HCC from NASH, another major factor contributing to cirrhosis. Due to the rising incidence of obesity, NASH has become a leading cause of cirrhosis around the world. Since 2010, the proportion of HCC caused by NASH has risen quickly, now accounting for 15–20% of cases in the Western world [6]. The proportion of metabolic syndrome and NASH attributable to the population is expected to exceed 20% due to the co-occurrence of these two disorders [37]. The incidence of HCC in NASH-associated cirrhosis (1–2% per year) is lower than in virus-related cirrhosis (3–5% per year), but it remains >1.1% per year, demonstrating that surveillance is cost-effective [38]. Several studies have shown that 25–30% of NASH-related HCC occurrences develop without cirrhosis, limiting the relevance of current surveillance programs that primarily target individuals with cirrhosis. However, the National Veterans Affairs Health System has discovered that the incidence of HCC annually is below the cost-effective threshold in people with non-cirrhotic NASH and surveillance should not be performed [38, 39].

9. Other risk factors

Many sociodemographic factors have been linked to HCC, particularly in individuals with cirrhosis. The risk of HCC increases with age, with those over 70 years of age showing the highest incidence [40]. HCC is also disproportionately male (male-to-female ratio of 2–3:1), which may reflect a clustering of risk factors among men, as well as differences in sex hormones [41]. HCC is more common in racial or ethnic minorities, particularly Hispanics, than in White people, according to studies. This disparity in prevalence could be related in part to the increased prevalence of single-nucleotide polymorphisms in PNPLA3, which are connected to NASH-associated HCC [42]. Smoking has also been linked to an increased risk of HCC in epidemiological studies [43]. Except for studies demonstrating a protective benefit of coffee and aspirin [44], the impact of diet in reducing the incidence of HCC is unknown.

10. Mechanisms/pathophysiology of HCC

HCC pathophysiology is a multistep process. The early stages of hepatocyte malignant transformation and HCC development are caused by the interaction of several variables. The cellular environment, immune cells, and the severity of chronic liver disease must all be considered, including genetic predisposition, and reciprocal interactions among viral and nonviral risk factors. From the early stages of transformation to invasion and then metastasis, the microenvironment plays an important role in cancer progression.

11. Origin of HCC cell

HCC's cell of origin is a point of contention. It is possible for liver cancer to originate from liver stem cells, transit-amplifying populations, or mature hepatocytes, just like in any other type of cancer. There is general controversy over whether liver stem cells exist and function. Additionally, mature hepatocytes have a high proliferation capacity after injury, which allows them to survive for long periods of time. Several studies on mouse models reported that HCC is believed to develop from transformed mature hepatocytes; however, other studies suggest HCC may originate from putative stem cells in the liver [45]. Intrahepatic cholangiocarcinomas and tumors with mixed HCC or cholangiocarcinoma form, on the other hand, often appear to emerge from adult hepatocytes, highlighting the principles of metaplasia and cell plasticity (i.e. trans-differentiation). These data back the idea that a tumor's form and epigenetic landscape may not always represent its cell of origin [46, 47].

12. Mutations of cancer-driver genes in HCC

High-throughput next-generation sequencing has identified cancer-driver genes recurrently changed in HCC with oncogenic or tumor-suppressive properties. In 80% of cases of HCC, driver gene alterations are found in the TERT promoter, chromosome translocations, telomerase activation, and gene amplification [7, 48]. Studies have shown that mutations in AXIN1 (inhibitors of the Wnt pathway), CTNNB1 (encoding-catenin), or APC (inhibitors of the Wnt pathway) inactivation activate the Wnt-β catenin signaling pathway in 30–50% of cases [7, 48]. CCNE1, TP53, ARID1A, RB1, CCNA2, PTEN, RPS6KA3, ARID2, and NFE2L2 are all known to have mutations or genetic changes that affect cell cycle control. AKT-mTOR and MAPK pathways, as well as genes involved in epigenetic regulation and oxidative stress, have been linked to HCC. AKT-mTOR and MAPK pathways, as well as genes involved in epigenetic regulation and oxidative stress, have been linked to HCC. The recurrent overexpression and activation of oncogenic signaling pathways, including receptor tyrosine kinases, are also linked to focal chromosomal amplification of MYC, CCND1, VEGFA, FGF19, and MET [49]. In spite of the fact that cancer-driver gene mutations can occur at random, certain genes seem to be associated with specific molecular HCC subclasses based on transcriptome profiles and histological phenotypes [8, 9, 50]. At least 20–25% of HCC patients have a potentially actionable mutation, according to current standards [7, 8, 51]. In the pathogenesis of HCC, it has been well documented that risk factors cooperate with cancer-driver mutations. In patients with a GSTT1 null mutation, for instance, the harmful effects of aflatoxin B1 are amplified by HBV infection [52, 53]. In addition, patients who use a lot of alcohol are more likely to have polymorphisms in PNPLA3, TM6SF2, and HSD17B13 [54, 55].

13. Molecular alterations associated with viral infection

The TERT promoter is the most common locus of HBV-mediated insertional mutagenesis, resulting in overexpression of telomerase, the enzyme responsible for telomere length maintenance [56]. Telomerase activation inhibits the chromosomal erosion that occurs naturally with each cell division as people age. Telomerase activity on the ectopic enhances cell transformation and protects cells against senescence [57]. Other HBV-associated recurrent insertions have been shown to activate potent oncogenes involved in cell cycle control, such as CCNA2 or CCNE1. Replicative stress and complex rearrangements are caused by these oncogenic changes throughout the genome [58]. Adeno-associated virus 2 (AAV2) showed identical insertional oncogenic mutagenesis in a small group of HCC patients, with a shared hot point of the viral insertion inside the TERT promoter, CCNA2, and CCNE1 [59]. These findings show that viral infection activates particular oncogenes, which act as early facilitators of hepatocyte transformation. HCV infection, on the other hand, has no direct carcinogenic effect, and the induction of mutations is driven by the oxidative stress caused by persistent inflammation.

14. Mutational signatures in HCC

Hepatocytes are subjected to multiple genetic mutations and epigenetic alterations throughout the progression of chronic liver disease and cirrhosis, which are the most common causes of HCC. Several risk factors that cause DNA changes are linked to particular mutational signatures during this process [7, 60]. In exome sequencing analyses of HCC, patients from Asia and Africa who had been exposed to aristolochic acid (A > T mutations in CTG trinucleotide) and aflatoxin B1 (C > A mutations) had mutational signatures 22 and 24, respectively [7, 61]. Mutations of the C > A at dinucleotide sequences in signature 4 were linked with tobacco smoking, while the T > C mutations at TpA dinucleotide in signature 16 were related to alcohol consumption [62]. It remains to be seen whether this discovery can be turned into preventative measures. It is well known that the liver is capable of detoxifying a variety of chemicals that may cause mutations in the hepatocyte genome, leading to the development of cancer.

15. Molecular classes of HCC

Several studies have created a molecular and immune categorization for HCC based on genomic, epigenomic, histopathological, and immunological analysis [1, 9, 63]. Molecular classes of HCC have been identified based on the principal molecular drivers and pathways involved [9, 63–67] or the tumor's immunology status [8, 68]. The molecular classifications are associated with specific genomic abnormalities, histological signatures, and clinical outcomes. Approximately half of all HCCs are of the proliferation type [49]. The proliferation type is characterized by mutations in TP53 and FGF19 or CCND1 amplification, and it is more common in HBV-associated cancers with poor prognosis. Within the proliferation class, there are two subclasses: proliferation progenitor cells and proliferation-Wnt-TGF cells. Twenty-five to thirty percent of HCC are proliferation-progenitor cells, which are characterized by activation of classical cell proliferation pathways, i.e. the expression of progenitor cell markers (such as EPCAM and FTP) is also related to the activation of signaling pathways (PI3K-AKT-mTOR, RAS-MAPK, and MET and IGF signaling cascades [49, 64]. In alcohol- and HCV-related HCC, non-proliferative tumors represent more than half of all cases; these tumors have better outcomes and correspond to TCGA cluster 2 [65]. Within the nonproliferative class, at least two distinct subgroups have been described: one with dominant canonical Wnt signaling and mutations in CTNNB1 [69] and the other with IFN signaling activation [49].

Reports on the classification of HCC based on immune cell status have added to the knowledge of HCC's molecular characteristics [68]. This categorization classifies HCC tumors into four subclasses: immunological-active, immune-exhausted, immune-intermediate, and immune-excluded, and gives additional information based on immune features. Immune cell infiltrations are categorized into two subclasses: immune-active and immune-exhausted. In HCC tumors that are immune-active, helper T (CD4+) and cytotoxic T (CD8+) cells are enriched and ICIs are effective. The depletion of CD8+ cells driven by TGF is prevalent in immune-exhausted tumors. In contrast, immune-excluded tumors lack T cell infiltrates and are characterized by a disproportionate increase in regulatory T cells (Tregs), as well as canonical Wnt signaling and other immune-suppressive pathways. Immune-excluded tumors often develop ICI resistance [70].

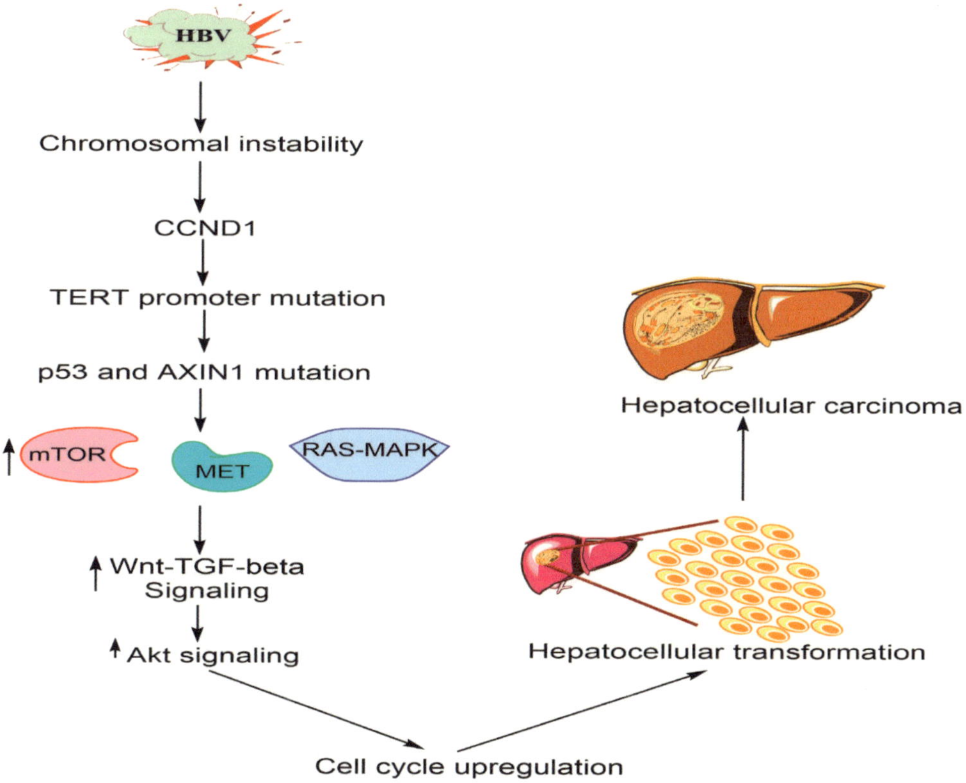

Figure 1.
The molecular mechanism of HBV-induced HCC.

Obesity has been related to a higher risk of cancer in a variety of organs [71]. Obesity can cause systemic alterations, such as impaired immune function and endocrine abnormalities, which are common in cancers of many types. According to current research, fatty liver disease is quickly becoming the primary cause of HCC in the Western world [6]. The effects of metabolic and oxidative stress, immune dysfunction, abnormal inflammatory responses, impaired endocrine, and adipokine signaling have all been identified as pathways by which NAFLD or NASH cause HCC (**Figure 1**) [72, 73].

Several classical cell proliferation pathways are activated in HBV-associated HCC tumors, including PI3K-AKT-mTOR, RAS-MAPK, MET, and Wnt-TGF. A high chromosomal instability level and frequent TP53 and AXIN1 mutations are additional features of HBV-induced HCC (**Figure 2**).

Nonalcoholic steatohepatitis (NASH), alcoholic steatohepatitis, and hepatitis C virus (HCV) infection promote the development of HCC tumors. Here, the risk factors cause chromosomal instability with frequent mutations in the TERT promoter

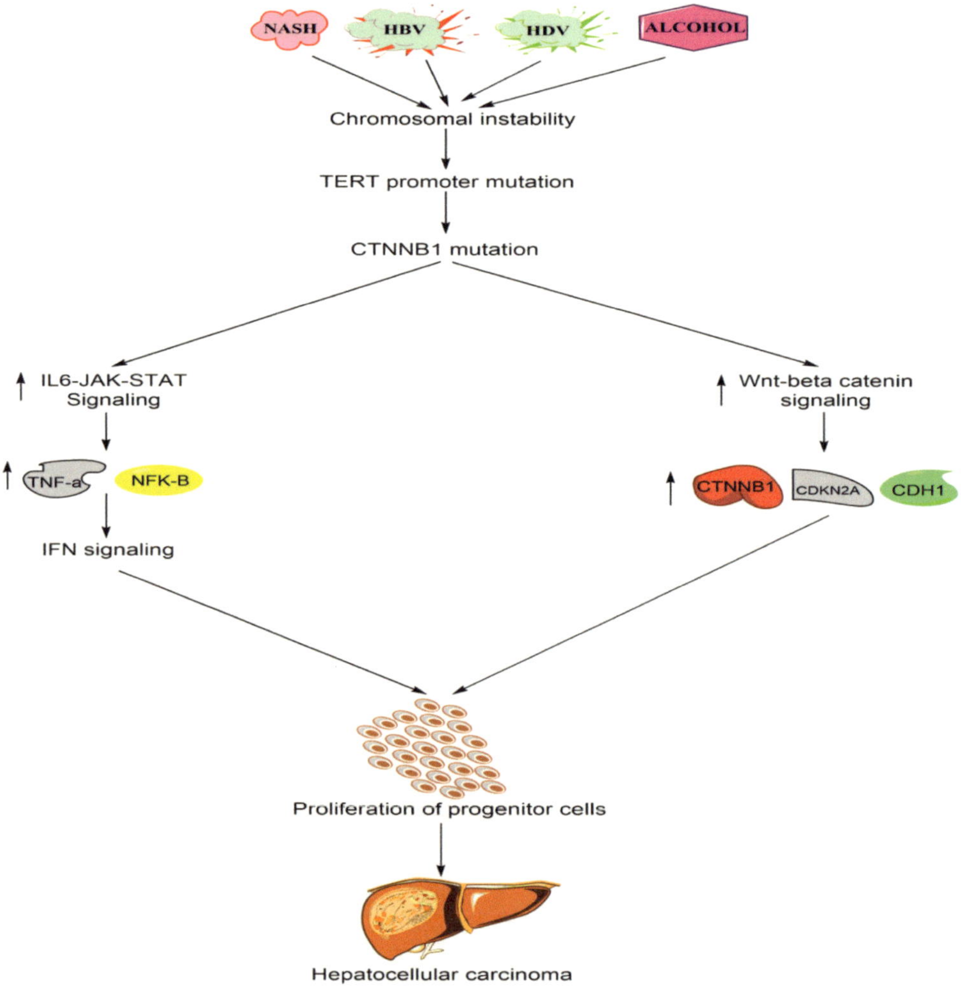

Figure 2.
The molecular pathogenesis of HCC induced by NASH, HCV, HDV, and alcohol.

sequence which, in turn, leads to the CTNNB1 mutations and activation of either WNT-β-catenin signaling pathway or IL6-JAK-STAT signaling pathway. The activation of either or both of these signaling pathway promote the proliferation of progenitor cells leading to an inflammatory tumor microenvironment and ultimately to HCC.

16. Oxidative stress and HCC

Fatty acid overload causes oxidative stress and endoplasmic reticulum (ER) stress in hepatocytes, resulting in pathological inflammation and cell death [72, 74]. HCC was induced in one study in mice following ER stress-induced inflammation via NF-κB and TNF-α signaling pathways [75]. These toxicological processes of HCC, however, are yet to be demonstrated in human. Hepatocytes with abnormal fatty acid metabolism are susceptible to DNA damage caused by reactive oxygen species (ROS) resulting from mitochondrial dysfunction [76]. Hepatocytes are also affected by changes in the expression of particular metabolic enzymes, which reduces their ability to repair DNA damage [77]. Changes in inflammatory signaling are also a result of the metabolic failure; for example, elevated levels of IL-17 (a tumor-promoting cytokine) have been seen in human NASH [78]. A number of pathogenic lipids are produced as oncometabolites in NASH in addition to increased lipid production [79, 80]. When mTORC2 is continuously activated in mouse hepatocytes, a high level of glucosylceramide is produced, increasing ROS production, which can lead to HCC [79]. Alterations in cholesterol metabolism may also have a role in HCC pathogenesis [80], possibly by causing the generation of pro-tumorigenic nuclear receptor ligands. Although autophagy has antitumor properties, one study found that lipophagy (autophagic destruction of lipid droplets) plays a crucial role in HCC progression. Hepatocytes from NASH patients and a mouse model of HCC overexpress sequestosome 1 (also called p62), a lipophagy regulator [81]. Patients with NASH had a higher risk of HCC than those with NAFLD according to studies [6]. In one experiment, fatty acid-induced oxidative stress in hepatocytes increased the expression of STAT1 and STAT3, two pro-inflammatory transcription factors that generally operate in tandem [82]. Surprisingly, a high level of STAT1 promoted NASH progression in this mouse model, while a high level of STAT3 promoted HCC, both independently [82]. Accordingly, similar inflammatory signals may promote progression from NAFLD to NASH or HCC in different ways. This is because NAFLD is more common in the general population than NASH [6]; the data indicate the need to understand how NAFLD, regardless of NASH, can lead to HCC. When hepatocytes are overloaded with fatty acids, the increased ER stress, pathological lipophagy, ROS generation, and a lowered reducing power (low NADH or NADPH levels) may combine to generate oncogenic genetic changes and accelerate the development of malignant cells.

Based on transcriptomic-based phenotypic classes, hepatocellular carcinoma (HCC) can be divided into two primary molecular groupings [49, 64–67]. More aggressive tumors with weak histological differentiation, high vascular invasion, and higher levels of alpha-fetoprotein (AFP) belong to the proliferation class [50]. In S1 or iCluster 3 [64, 65], Wnt-TGF activation leads to an immune-exhausted phenotype [68], while in S2 or iCluster 1 [64, 65], stem cells markers (CK19, EPCAM) as well as IGF2 and EPCAM signaling pathways are expressed [50]. In hepatitis B virus (HBV)-associated tumors, cell proliferation pathways such as PI3K-AKT-mTOR, RAS-MAPK, MET, and IGF are usually activated. Furthermore, numerous TP53 mutations, high chromosomal instability, and widespread DNA hypomethylation are also characteristics of this group. The nonproliferation class consists of tumors that are less aggressive, well-differentiated histologically, have low AFP levels, and have fewer vascular invasions [50]. These tumors can be caused by nonalcoholic steatohepatitis (NASH), alcoholic steatohepatitis (ASH), or infection with hepatitis C virus (HCV) [49, 64–67]. This class is divided into two distinct subgroups: the WNT—catenin CTNNB1 subclass has frequent CTNNB1 mutations and activated WNT—catenin signaling, leading to an immune-excluded phenotype with low immune infiltration [49, 67, 68]; and the interferon subclass has a highly activated IL6-JAK-STAT signaling pathway, leading to a more inflamed microtumor with many TERT promoter mutations, and this class has chromosomal stability [63–68].

17. Immune infiltration of fatty liver

The histological characteristic of NASH is immune cell infiltration of the obese liver [72]. The establishment of animal models that accurately reproduce human HCC is critical for basic pathogenesis research as well as translational research [83–97]. Immune cells and cytokines have been found to have an essential role in the pathogenesis of HCC in several experimental types. In mouse models, for example, persistent NASH causes CD8+ T cell activation, which leads to hepatocyte destruction and HCC [98]. As a consequence of NAFLD, intrahepatic CD4+ T cells are selectively depleted, which are necessary to initiate an effective adaptive immune response against tumors [99]. Additionally, B cells, Treg cells, natural killer cells, and other myeloid cells have been associated with NASH-induced HCC [72, 73]. The activation and recruitment of platelets in the liver also contribute to HCC formation in mice, specifically via platelet glycoprotein Ib (GPIb) signaling, which is in line with clinical data [100], implying that this pathway has the therapeutic potential [101]. The causal function of NASH in HCC was also linked to a changed cytokine milieu [74]. NASH, for example, has been demonstrated to overexpress hepatic IL-6 and TNF-α, which are both causes of HCC in various etiologies [102].

On the background of fatty liver disease, all of the mechanisms described earlier could promote HCC at the same time. Their relative involvement to human HCC, however, is uncertain at this time. The comparison of mutational signatures in NASH-associated HCC versus HCC from other causes should aid in determining the relative contributions of different variables.

18. Inflammation and HCC

HCC is an archetypal inflammation-related malignancy, with chronic inflammation caused by viral hepatitis, excessive alcohol consumption, NAFLD, or NASH accounting for 90% of the HCC burden. In the development of HCC [103], the immunological microenvironment plays a critical role. Immune infiltrates are associated with a better prognosis in HCC, possibly due to more effective antitumor immunity [68, 104]. Immune signals such as IL-6, lymphotoxin-, and TNF-α have been shown to accelerate hepatocarcinogenesis and impact tumor aggressiveness in mouse models of HCC [47, 105], yet immune responses can also slow the course of liver cancer [103]. In addition, the liver has the greatest number of immune cells in the body and has a unique immunological state that allows it to survive the constant influx of inflammatory signals coming from the gut [103]. Understanding this specific hepatic immune system is likely important given the intricate interplay between malignant hepatocytes and the liver immune system [103, 106]. A surprising finding in mice and humans is that VEGF released by malignant hepatocytes creates an immune-tolerant, pro-tumorigenic microenvironment [49, 107], suggesting that inhibiting the VEGF cascade might have a positive effect on liver immunity by modifying VEGF production. Interestingly, the combination of ICIs and certain targeted medicines such as VEGF inhibitors had greater survival advantages than the use of single agents [16, 108].

It has been shown that hepatocytes in chronically inflamed livers interact with numerous cell types including macrophages, endothelial cells, stellate cells, and various types of lymphocytes [103, 106]. Due to its importance in immuno-oncology therapy, researchers are paying more attention to the adaptive immune system's involvement. Mouse models have revealed that practically every immune cell type can play both pro-tumor and antitumor roles [103]. In addition to producing pro-tumorigenic cytokines and growth factors that support tumor cell proliferation or inhibit apoptosis, immune cells also diminish nearby lymphocytes' antitumorigenic function. The NF-B and JAK-STAT pathways have been identified as major inflammatory signaling pathways implicated in the promotion of HCC in studies [109], and this assertion was confirmed in a transcriptomic analysis of human HCC [110]. Immune monitoring and the destruction of premalignant or completely changed malignant hepatocytes are the adaptive immune system's main antitumor functions [104].

19. The role of adaptive immune system in HCC

The main effectors of antitumor immunity are cytotoxic T (CD8+) cells. As a result, one study found that depleting these T cells in mice increased HCC burden [111], while another found that these T cells promote premalignant hepatocyte surveillance [112]. Several studies in mice have shown that the depletion of CD8+ T cells can also reduce tumor burden [98]. Analyses of human HCC samples suggest that some individuals have functional CD8+ T lymphocytes that produce antitumor effector molecules such as granzyme A, granzyme B, and perforin [113]. However, single-cell sequencing of human HCC T cells has revealed that the CD8+ T cells are often dysfunctional in HCC [114]. There is no clear understanding of the causes of CD8+ T cell dysfunction, which leads to diminished proliferation and the inability to generate cytotoxic effector molecules. Increasing numbers of Treg cells within the tumor are linked with poorer clinical outcomes in HCC, and Treg cells are thought to be a primary cause of T cell dysfunction [115]. Treg cells' immunosuppressive capabilities may be mediated by CD10 and TGF116 production, suggesting that blocking these cytokines could make HCC more susceptible to ICIs. HCC-infiltrating Treg cells are known to suppress immune responses through the hyaluronic acid receptor, layilin, which is interesting [116]. As a result of a layilin induction, CD8+ T cells exhibited dysfunction in human HCC, and layilin overexpression was associated with distinct mRNA expression signatures in lymphocytes [114].

Although B cells were once assumed to be innocent bystanders in cancer, new data suggest that they have an active role in the adaptive immune system's interaction with cancer [117]. B lymphocytes both stimulated and inhibited tumor growth in mice models of HCC [118]. Furthermore, one study found that IgA-expressing cells actively suppressed CD8+ T cell activity, which aided HCC growth [111]. Furthermore, studies in humans and mice have shown that tertiary lymphoid structures, which are crucial for adaptive immune responses to cancer [119], have both pro-tumor and antitumor capacity in HCC [120, 121].

20. The microenvironment of cirrhosis in HCC

The risk of HCC is high enough to warrant surveillance once the patient has reached cirrhosis, even though some etiologies (for instance, HCV versus autoimmune hepatitis) are more likely to cause HCC than others [10, 11]. In response to chronic injury, hepatic stellate cells play an important role [122]. Upon activation, it undergoes phenotypic changes and synthesizes components of the extracellular matrix, mainly collagen, as well as growth factors, which promote neoangiogenesis, endothelial cell migration, and fibrosis [123]. Cirrhosis and portal hypertension have a histological substrate in which the hepatic architecture is distorted and the vasculature is disordered. Premalignant senescent hepatocytes respond to this condition by secreting chemokines that impair senescent surveillance and immune-mediated tumor suppression in vivo [112]. Experimental models have also demonstrated that CD4+ cells are relevant in promoting NAFLD-related HCC [99], and the interaction between the innate immune system and the intestinal microbiota plays a role in promoting the development of HCC [124, 125]. In HCC, the immune system, in addition to fibrosis, plays a significant role in the cancer field effect. The cancer field effect refers to the favorable microenvironment in cirrhosis that favors tumor formation. The primary molecular elements unregulated in this microenvironment have been identified through various genomic investigations. Several gene profiles obtained from cirrhotic tissue are associated with the probability of developing HCC and can be utilized to risk stratify patients [110, 126, 127]. The presence of these gene signatures is associated with cancer risk, the incidence of hepatic decompensation in patients, and overall survival [126, 127]. More research has been done on the genetic characteristics of the cirrhosis inflammatory milieu that contribute to HCC development [128]. In 50% of neighboring cirrhotic tissue from HCC patients, an immune-mediated cancer field molecular subclass was observed. In addition to lymphocyte infiltration, this subclass can be further divided based on pro-inflammatory or immunosuppressive signal activation. In the immunosuppressive subclass, which accounted for 10% of patients and had a threefold higher risk of developing HCC, TGF signaling, T-cell exhaustion, and overexpression of immunological checkpoints (such as CTLA4, TIGIT, and LAG3) were shown to be more prevalent [128]. Modulating the tumor microenvironment's role in HCC's natural history would be a compelling reason for altering the dynamic crosstalk between hepatocytes and the hepatic immune system [103].

Author details

Rahmat Adetutu Adisa[1*] and Lateef Adegboyega Sulaimon[1,2]

1 Faculty of Basic Medical Sciences, Department of Biochemistry, Laboratory for Biomembranes, Toxicology and Cancer Research, College of Medicine, University of Lagos, Lagos, Nigeria

2 Department of Chemical Sciences, College of Natural and Applied Sciences, Crescent University, Abeokuta, Ogun State, Nigeria

*Address all correspondence to: radisa@unilag.edu.ng

References

[1] Llovet JM et al. Hepatocellular carcinoma. Nature Reviews Diseases Primers. 2016;**2**:16018

[2] Villanueva A. Hepatocellular carcinoma. The New England Journal of Medicine. 2019;**380**:1450-1462

[3] International Agency for Research on Cancer. GLOBOCAN 2018. IARC. 2020. Available from: https://gco.iarc.fr/today/online-analysis-map?v=2020&mode=population&mode_population=continents&population=900&populations=900&key=asr&sex=0&cancer=11&type=0&statistic=5&prevalence=0&population_groupearth&color_palette=default&map_scale=quantile&map_nb_colors=5&continent=0&rotate=%255B10%252C0%255D

[4] Akinyemiju T et al. The burden of primary liver cancer and underlying etiologies from 1990 to 2015 at the global, regional, and national level. JAMA Oncology. 2017;**3**:1683

[5] Kanwal F et al. Risk of hepatocellular cancer in HCV patients treated with direct- acting antiviral agents. Gastroenterology. 2017;**153**:996-1005

[6] Estes C, Razavi H, Loomba R, Younossi Z, Sanyal AJ. Modeling the epidemic of nonalcoholic fatty liver disease demonstrates an exponential increase in burden of disease. Hepatology. 2018;**67**:123-133

[7] Schulze K et al. Exome sequencing of hepatocellular carcinomas identifies new mutational signatures and potential therapeutic targets. Nature Genetics. 2015;**47**:505-511

[8] Llovet JM, Montal R, Sia D, Finn RS. Molecular therapies and precision medicine for hepatocellular carcinoma. Nature Reviews: Clinical Oncology. 2018;**15**:599-616

[9] Zucman- Rossi J, Villanueva A, Nault J-C, Llovet JM. Genetic landscape and biomarkers of hepatocellular carcinoma. Gastroenterology. 2015;**149**:1226-1239

[10] European Association for the Study of the Liver. EASL clinical practice guidelines: Management of hepatocellular carcinoma. Journal of Hepatology. 2018;**69**:182-236

[11] Marrero JA et al. Diagnosis, staging, and management of hepatocellular carcinoma: 2018 practice guidance by the American Association for the Study of Liver Diseases. Hepatology. 2018;**68**:723-750

[12] Llovet JM, De Baere T, Kulik L, Haber PK, Greten TF, Meyer T, et al. Locoregional therapies in the era of molecular and immune treatments for hepatocellular carcinoma. Nature Reviews Gastroenterology and Hepatology. 2021;**18**(5):293-313. DOI: 10.1038/s41575-020-00395-0

[13] Tabrizian P et al. A US multicenter analysis of 2529 HCC patients undergoing liver transplantation: 10-year outcome assessing the role of down-staging to within Milan criteria [abstract 15]. Hepatology. 2019;**70**:10-11

[14] Llovet J, Bruix J. Systematic review of randomized trials for unresectable hepatocellular carcinoma: Chemoembolization improves survival. Hepatology. 2003;**37**:429-442

[15] Salem R et al. Y90 radioembolization significantly prolongs time to progression compared with

chemoembolization in patients with hepatocellular carcinoma. Gastroenterology. 2016;**151**:1155-1163

[16] Finn RS et al. Atezolizumab plus bevacizumab in unresectable hepatocellular carcinoma. The New England Journal of Medicine. 2020;**382**:1894-1905

[17] Llovet JM et al. Sorafenib in advanced hepatocellular carcinoma. The New England Journal of Medicine. 2008;**359**:378-390

[18] Kudo M et al. Lenvatinib versus sorafenib in first- line treatment of patients with unresectable hepatocellular carcinoma: A randomized phase 3 non- inferiority trial. Lancet. 2018;**391**:1163-1173

[19] Bruix J et al. Regorafenib for patients with hepatocellular carcinoma who progressed on sorafenib treatment (RESORCE): A randomised, double-blind, placebo- controlled, phase 3 trial. Lancet. 2017;**389**:56-66

[20] Abou- Alfa GK et al. Cabozantinib in patients with advanced and progressing hepatocellular carcinoma. The New England Journal of Medicine. 2018;**379**:54-63

[21] Zhu AX et al. Ramucirumab after sorafenib in patients with advanced hepatocellular carcinoma and increased α- fetoprotein concentrations (REACH-2): A randomized, double- blind, placebo-controlled, phase 3 trial. The Lancet Oncology. 2019;**20**:282-296

[22] El- Khoueiry AB et al. Nivolumab in patients with advanced hepatocellular carcinoma (CheckMate 040): An open-label, non- comparative, phase 1/2 dose escalation and expansion trial. Lancet. 2017;**389**:2492-2502

[23] Finn RS et al. Pembrolizumab as second- line therapy in patients with advanced hepatocellular carcinoma in KEYNOTE-240: A randomized, double-blind, phase III trial. Journal of Clinical Oncology. 2020;**38**:193-202

[24] McGlynn KA, Petrick JL, London WT. Global epidemiology of hepatocellular carcinoma: An emphasis on demographic and regional variability. Clinics in Liver Disease. 2015;**19**:223-238

[25] Rahib L et al. Projecting cancer incidence and deaths to 2030: The unexpected burden of thyroid, liver, and pancreas cancers in the United States. Cancer Research. 2014;**74**:2913-2921

[26] Trinchet J-C et al. Complications and competing risks of death in compensated viral cirrhosis (ANRS CO12 CirVir prospective cohort). Hepatology. 2015;**62**:737-750

[27] Fracanzani A. Increased cancer risk in a cohort of 230 patients with hereditary hemochromatosis in comparison to matched control patients with non–iron- related chronic liver disease. Hepatology. 2001;**33**:647-651

[28] Wang J, Chenivesse X, Henglein B, Bréchot C. Hepatitis B virus integration in a cyclin A gene in a hepatocellular carcinoma. Nature. 1990;**343**:555-557

[29] Kew MC. Synergistic interaction between aflatoxin B1 and hepatitis B virus in hepatocarcinogenesis. Liver International. 2003;**23**:405-409

[30] Chang MH et al. Long- term effects of hepatitis B immunization of infants in preventing liver cancer. Gastroenterology. 2016;**151**:472-480

[31] Jain MK et al. Evaluation of a multifaceted intervention to reduce health disparities in hepatitis C screening:

A pre- post analysis. Hepatology. 2019;**70**:40-50

[32] Ioannou GN et al. Increased risk for hepatocellular carcinoma persists up to 10 years after HCV eradication in patients with baseline cirrhosis or high FIB-4 scores. Gastroenterology. 2019;**157**:1264-1278

[33] Llovet JM, Villanueva A. Effect of HCV clearance with direct- acting antiviral agents on HCC. Nature Reviews. Gastroenterology & Hepatology. 2016;**13**:561-562

[34] Puigvehí M, Moctezuma-Velázquez C, Villanueva A, Llovet JM. The oncogenic role of hepatitis delta virus in hepatocellular carcinoma. JHEP Reports. 2019;**1**:120-130

[35] Jepsen P, Ott P, Andersen PK, Sørensen HT, Vilstrup H. Risk for hepatocellular carcinoma in patients with alcoholic cirrhosis. Annals of Internal Medicine. 2012;**156**:841

[36] Lin C-W et al. Heavy alcohol consumption increases the incidence of hepatocellular carcinoma in hepatitis B virus-related cirrhosis. Journal of Hepatology. 2013;**58**:730-735. DOI: 10.1016/j.jhep.2012.11.045

[37] Welzel TM et al. Population-attributable fractions of risk factors for hepatocellular carcinoma in the United States. The American Journal of Gastroenterology. 2013;**108**:1314-1321

[38] Kanwal F et al. Risk of hepatocellular cancer in patients with non- alcoholic fatty liver disease. Gastroenterology. 2018;**155**:1828-1837

[39] Mittal S et al. Hepatocellular carcinoma in the absence of cirrhosis in United States veterans is associated with nonalcoholic fatty liver disease. Clinical Gastroenterology and Hepatology. 2016;**14**:124-131

[40] Rich NE, Yopp AC, Singal AG, Murphy CC. Hepatocellular carcinoma incidence is decreasing among younger adults in the United States. Clinical Gastroenterology and Hepatology. 2020;**18**:242-248

[41] Bray F et al. Global cancer statistics 2018: GLOBOCAN estimates of incidence and mortality worldwide for 36 cancers in 185 countries. CA: A Cancer Journal for Clinicians. 2018;**68**:394-424

[42] Rich NE et al. Racial and ethnic differences in presentation and outcomes of hepatocellular carcinoma. Clinical Gastroenterology and Hepatology. 2019;**17**:551-559

[43] Lee Y-CA et al. Meta- analysis of epidemiologic studies on cigarette smoking and liver cancer. International Journal of Epidemiology. 2009;**38**:1497-1511

[44] Bravi F, Bosetti C, Tavani A, Gallus S, La Vecchia C. Coffee reduces risk for hepatocellular carcinoma: An updated meta- analysis. Clinical Gastroenterology and Hepatology. 2013;**11**:1413-1421

[45] Sia D, Villanueva A, Friedman SL, Llovet JM. Liver cancer cell of origin, molecular class, and effects on patient prognosis. Gastroenterology. 2017;**152**:745-761

[46] Pikarsky E. Neighbourhood deaths cause a switch in cancer subtype. Nature. 2018;**562**:45-46

[47] Seehawer M et al. Necroptosis microenvironment directs lineage commitment in liver cancer. Nature. 2018;**562**:69-75

[48] Guichard C et al. Integrated analysis of somatic mutations and focal copy-number changes identifies key genes and pathways in hepatocellular carcinoma. Nature Genetics. 2012;**44**:694-698

[49] Chiang DY et al. Focal gains of VEGFA and molecular classification of hepatocellular carcinoma. Cancer Research. 2008;**68**:6779-6788

[50] Calderaro J, Ziol M, Paradis V, Zucman- Rossi J. Molecular and histological correlations in liver cancer. Journal of Hepatology. 2019;**71**:616-630

[51] Hyman DM, Taylor BS, Baselga J. Implementing genome- driven oncology. Cell. 2017;**168**:584-599

[52] Bressac B, Kew M, Wands J, Ozturk M. Selective G to T mutations of p53 gene in hepatocellular carcinoma from southern Africa. Nature. 1991;**350**:429-431

[53] Wang B et al. Null genotypes of GSTM1 and GSTT1 contribute to hepatocellular carcinoma risk: Evidence from an updated meta- analysis. Journal of Hepatology. 2010;**53**:508-518

[54] Romeo S et al. Genetic variation in PNPLA3 confers susceptibility to nonalcoholic fatty liver disease. Nature Genetics. 2008;**40**:1461-1465

[55] Buch S et al. A genome- wide association study confirms PNPLA3 and identifies TM6SF2 and MBOAT7 as risk loci for alcohol- related cirrhosis. Nature Genetics. 2015;**47**:1443-1448

[56] Paterlini- Bréchot P et al. Hepatitis B virus- related insertional mutagenesis occurs frequently in human liver cancers and recurrently targets human telomerase gene. Oncogene. 2003;**22**:3911-3916

[57] Nault J-C, Ningarhari M, Rebouissou S, Zucman- Rossi J. The role of telomeres and telomerase in cirrhosis and liver cancer. Nature Reviews. Gastroenterology & Hepatology. 2019;**16**:544-558

[58] Bayard Q et al. Cyclin A2/E1 activation defines a hepatocellular carcinoma subclass with a rearrangement signature of replication stress. Nature Communications. 2018;**9**:5235

[59] Nault J-C et al. Recurrent AAV2-related insertional mutagenesis in human hepatocellular carcinomas. Nature Genetics. 2015;**47**:1187-1193

[60] Letouzé E et al. Mutational signatures reveal the dynamic interplay of risk factors and cellular processes during liver tumorigenesis. Nature Communications. 2017;**8**:1315

[61] Ng AWT et al. Aristolochic acids and their derivatives are widely implicated in liver cancers in Taiwan and throughout Asia. Science Translational Medicine. 2017;**9**:eaan6446

[62] Alexandrov LB et al. Signatures of mutational processes in human cancer. Nature. 2013;**500**:415-421

[63] Rebouissou S, Nault J-C. Advances in molecular classification and precision oncology in hepatocellular carcinoma. Journal of Hepatology. 2020;**72**:215-229

[64] Hoshida Y et al. Integrative transcriptome analysis reveals common molecular subclasses of human hepatocellular carcinoma. Cancer Research. 2009;**69**:7385-7392

[65] Cancer Genome Atlas Research Network. Comprehensive and integrative genomic characterization of hepatocellular carcinoma. Cell. 2017;**169**:1327-1341

[66] Lee J-S et al. A novel prognostic subtype of human hepatocellular carcinoma derived from hepatic progenitor cells. Nature Medicine. 2006;**12**:410-416

[67] Boyault S et al. Transcriptome classification of HCC is related to gene alterations and to new therapeutic targets. Hepatology. 2007;**45**:42-52

[68] Sia D et al. Identification of an immune- specific class of hepatocellular carcinoma, based on molecular features. Gastroenterology. 2017;**153**:812-826

[69] Lachenmayer A et al. Wnt-pathway activation in two molecular classes of hepatocellular carcinoma and experimental modulation by sorafenib. Clinical Cancer Research. 2012;**18**:4997-5007

[70] Ruiz de Galarreta, M. et al. β-Catenin activation promotes immune escape and resistance to anti- PD-1 therapy in hepatocellular carcinoma. Cancer Discovery 9, 1124-1141 (2019).

[71] Renehan AG, Tyson M, Egger M, Heller RF, Zwahlen M. Body- mass index and incidence of cancer: A systematic review and meta- analysis of prospective observational studies. Lancet. 2008;**371**:569-578

[72] Anstee QM, Reeves HL, Kotsiliti E, Govaere O, Heikenwalder M. From NASH to HCC: Current concepts and future challenges. Nature Reviews. Gastroenterology & Hepatology. 2019;**16**:411-428

[73] Sutti S, Albano E. Adaptive immunity: An emerging player in the progression of NAFLD. Nature Reviews. Gastroenterology & Hepatology. 2020;**17**:81-92

[74] Friedman SL, Neuschwander-Tetri BA, Rinella M, Sanyal AJ. Mechanisms of NAFLD development and therapeutic strategies. Nature Medicine. 2018;**24**:908-922

[75] Nakagawa H et al. ER stress cooperates with hypernutrition to trigger TNF-A – dependent spontaneous HCC development. Cancer Cell. 2014;**26**:331-343

[76] Nishida N et al. Unique features associated with hepatic oxidative DNA damage and DNA methylation in non-alcoholic fatty liver disease. Journal of Gastroenterology and Hepatology. 2016;**31**:1646-1653

[77] Tummala KS et al. Inhibition of de novo NAD+ synthesis by oncogenic URI causes liver tumorigenesis through DNA damage. Cancer Cell. 2014;**26**:826-839

[78] Gomes AL et al. Metabolic inflammation- associated IL-17A causes non- alcoholic steatohepatitis and hepatocellular carcinoma. Cancer Cell. 2016;**30**:161-175

[79] Guri Y et al. mTORC2 promotes tumorigenesis via lipid synthesis. Cancer Cell. 2017;**32**:807-823

[80] Liu D et al. Squalene epoxidase drives NAFLD- induced hepatocellular carcinoma and is a pharmaceutical target. Science Translational Medicine. 2018;**10**:eaap9840

[81] Umemura A et al. p62, upregulated during preneoplasia, induces hepatocellular carcinogenesis by maintaining survival of stressed HCC- initiating cells. Cancer Cell. 2016;**29**:935-948

[82] Grohmann M et al. Obesity drives STAT-1-dependent NASH and STAT-3-dependent HCC. Cell. 2018;**175**:1289-1306

[83] Henderson JM, Zhang HE, Polak N, Gorrell MD. Hepatocellular carcinoma: Mouse models and the potential roles of proteases. Cancer Letters. 2017;**387**:106-113

[84] Negro F. Natural history of NASH and HCC. Liver International. 2020;**40**:72-76

[85] Rudalska R et al. In vivo RNAi screening identifies a mechanism of sorafenib resistance in liver cancer. Nature Medicine. 2014;**20**:1138-1146

[86] Martinez- Quetglas I et al. IGF2 is up- regulated by epigenetic mechanisms in hepatocellular carcinomas and is an actionable oncogene product in experimental models. Gastroenterology. 2016;**151**:1192-1205

[87] Doudna JA, Charpentier E. The new frontier of genome engineering with CRISPR- Cas9. Science. 2014;**346**:1258096

[88] Cook N, Jodrell DI, Tuveson DA. Predictive in vivo animal models and translation to clinical trials. Drug Discovery Today. 2012;**17**:253-260

[89] Singh M, Ferrara N. Modeling and predicting clinical efficacy for drugs targeting the tumor milieu. Nature Biotechnology. 2012;**30**:648-657

[90] Newell P, Villanueva A, Friedman SL, Koike K, Llovet JM. Experimental models of hepatocellular carcinoma. Journal of Hepatology. 2008;**48**:858-879

[91] Bresnahan E, Ramadori P, Heikenwalder M, Zender L, Lujambio A. Novel patient- derived preclinical models of liver cancer. Journal of Hepatology. 2020;**72**:239-249

[92] Moriya K et al. The core protein of hepatitis C virus induces hepatocellular carcinoma in transgenic mice. Nature Medicine. 1998;**4**:1065-1067

[93] Hagel M et al. First selective small molecule inhibitor of FGFR4 for the treatment of hepatocellular carcinomas with an activated FGFR4 signaling pathway. Cancer Discovery. 2015;**5**:424-437

[94] Day C-P, Merlino G, Van Dyke T. Preclinical mouse cancer models: A maze of opportunities and challenges. Cell. 2015;**163**:39-53

[95] Jayson G, Harris J. How participants in cancer trials are chosen: Ethics and conflicting interests. Nature Reviews: Cancer. 2006;**6**:330-336

[96] Febbraio MA et al. Preclinical models for studying NASH- driven HCC: How useful are they? Cell Metabolism. 2019;**29**:18-26

[97] Sharpless NE, DePinho RA. The mighty mouse: Genetically engineered mouse models in cancer drug development. Nature Reviews: Drug Discovery. 2006;**5**:741-754

[98] Wolf MJ et al. Metabolic activation of intrahepatic CD8+ T cells and NKT cells causes nonalcoholic steatohepatitis and liver cancer via cross- talk with hepatocytes. Cancer Cell. 2014;**26**:549-564

[99] Ma C et al. NAFLD causes selective CD4+ T lymphocyte loss and promotes hepatocarcinogenesis. Nature. 2016;**531**:253-257

[100] Simon TG et al. Association of aspirin with hepatocellular carcinoma and liver- related mortality. The New England Journal of Medicine. 2020;**382**:1018-1028

[101] Malehmir M et al. Platelet GPIbα is a mediator and potential interventional

target for NASH and subsequent liver cancer. Nature Medicine. 2019;**25**:641-655

[102] Park EJ et al. Dietary and genetic obesity promote liver inflammation and tumorigenesis by enhancing IL-6 and TNF-A expression. Cell. 2010;**140**:197-208

[103] Ringelhan M, Pfister D, O'Connor T, Pikarsky E, Heikenwalder M. The immunology of hepatocellular carcinoma. Nature Immunology. 2018;**19**:222-232

[104] Wada Y, Nakashima O, Kutami R, Yamamoto O, Kojiro M. Clinicopathological study on hepatocellular carcinoma with lymphocytic infiltration. Hepatology. 1998;**27**:407-414

[105] Yuan D et al. Kupffer cell- derived TNF-A triggers cholangiocellular tumorigenesis through JNK due to chronic mitochondrial dysfunction and ROS. Cancer Cell. 2017;**31**:771-789

[106] Crispe IN. The liver as a lymphoid organ. Annual Review of Immunology. 2009;**27**:147-163

[107] Horwitz E et al. Human and mouse VEGFA- amplified hepatocellular carcinomas are highly sensitive to Sorafenib treatment. Cancer Discovery. 2014;**4**:730-743

[108] Finn RS et al. Phase Ib study of lenvatinib plus pembrolizumab in patients with unresectable hepatocellular carcinoma. Journal of Clinical Oncology. 2020;**38**:2960-2970

[109] Hou J, Zhang H, Sun B, Karin M. The immunobiology of hepatocellular carcinoma in humans and mice: Basic concepts and therapeutic implications. Journal of Hepatology. 2020;**72**:167-182

[110] Hoshida Y et al. Gene expression in fixed tissues and outcome in hepatocellular carcinoma. The New England Journal of Medicine. 2008;**359**:1995-2004

[111] Shalapour S et al. Inflammation-induced IgA+ cells dismantle anti- liver cancer immunity. Nature. 2017;**551**:340-345

[112] Kang TW et al. Senescence surveillance of pre- malignant hepatocytes limits liver cancer development. Nature. 2011;**479**:547-551

[113] Flecken T et al. Immunodominance and functional alterations of tumor-associated antigen- specific CD8+ T- cell responses in hepatocellular carcinoma. Hepatology. 2014;**59**:1415-1426

[114] Zheng C et al. Landscape of infiltrating T cells in liver cancer revealed by single- cell sequencing. Cell. 2017;**169**:1342-1356

[115] Langhans B et al. Role of regulatory T cells and checkpoint inhibition in hepatocellular carcinoma. Cancer Immunology, Immunotherapy. 2019;**68**:2055-2066

[116] Garnelo M et al. Interaction between tumour-infiltrating B cells and T cells controls the progression of hepatocellular carcinoma. Gut. 2017;**66**:342-351

[117] Bruno T. New predictors for immunotherapy responses sharpen our view of the tumour microenvironment. Nature. 2020;**577**:474-476

[118] Schneider C et al. Adaptive immunity suppresses formation and progression of diethylnitrosamine-induced liver cancer. Gut. 2012;**61**: 1733-1743

[119] Sautès- Fridman C, Petitprez F, Calderaro J, Fridman WH. Tertiary lymphoid structures in the era of cancer immunotherapy. Nature Reviews. Cancer. 2019;**19**:307-325

[120] Calderaro J et al. Intra- tumoral tertiary lymphoid structures are associated with a low risk of early recurrence of hepatocellular carcinoma. Journal of Hepatology. 2019;**70**:58-65

[121] Finkin S et al. Ectopic lymphoid structures function as microniches for tumor progenitor cells in hepatocellular carcinoma. Nature Immunology. 2015;**16**:1235-1244

[122] Tsuchida T, Friedman SL. Mechanisms of hepatic stellate cell activation. Nature Reviews. Gastroenterology & Hepatology. 2017;**14**:397-411

[123] Higashi T, Friedman SL, Hoshida Y. Hepatic stellate cells as key target in liver fibrosis. Advanced Drug Delivery Reviews. 2017;**121**:27-42

[124] Dapito DH et al. Promotion of hepatocellular carcinoma by the intestinal microbiota and TLR4. Cancer Cell. 2012;**21**:504-516

[125] Ma C et al. Gut microbiome-mediated bile acid metabolism regulates liver cancer via NKT cells. Science. 2018;**360**:eaan5931

[126] Hoshida Y et al. Prognostic gene expression signature for patients with hepatitis C–related early stage cirrhosis. Gastroenterology. 2013;**144**:1024-1030

[127] Budhu A et al. Prediction of venous metastases, recurrence, and prognosis in hepatocellular carcinoma based on a unique immune response signature of the liver microenvironment. Cancer Cell. 2006;**10**:99-111

[128] Moeini A et al. An immune gene expression signature associated with development of human hepatocellular carcinoma identifies mice that respond to chemopreventive agents. Gastroenterology. 2019;**157**:1383-1397